# M. GEESCOGE

# FROM MAN TO MEN

## Tips and Cases for Men to Better Know and Understand Women.

# FROM MAN TO MEN

Author: M. GEESCOGE

# IMPORTANT:

This book is not dedicated to the female audience.
However, it is not prohibited to read it.
Therefore, if any woman is curious
to know about this work,
please start from the
note that follows
immediately
below.

Thank you!

# AUTHOR'S NOTE

I don't want to seem derogatory towards the female audience by speaking so openly about women as I do here. On the contrary, my goal is to make men reflect on themselves and, within this reflection, seek to understand and accept women in all respects, in order to give them the best of themselves and what they always deserve, even though they often lack:
**love, attention, and understanding!**

# FROM MAN TO MEN

By: M. GEESCOGE

*"Every man has a thought,
every human being, a madness.
Every woman, a feminine air, and
every rule, of course, has an exception."*
*Aniel dos Santos (Diversities - 1985)*

## INTRODUCTION

For a long time, in conversations with friends, someone always asked me to write something that could guide men in their romantic relationships, with family, at work, with friends, in short, something that was truly dedicated to men. Faced with all that I always heard, one day I started feeding my mind and thinking about what I could write. The result was a deep dive into events, many of them significant in my life, and many others that marked the lives of my friends and colleagues. Others from people who simply stimulated my knowledge with stories of moments from their lives. And so on...

I want to clarify that the events portrayed here will not follow any order and will not have semantic rigidity. Often, the language may be colloquial, regional, and, therefore, not very committed to grammar itself. The names that may appear in the context will be imaginary, and no matter how much someone wants, the source and who the actual agent of the event is will not be revealed. I refer to you, therefore, with all the clarity and truth of each particularity focused here. And I say, to reinforce that nothing, except the names of the people, is a product of imagination. Everything happened at some point, whether with me, with friends, or with people who had the courage and confidence to one day tell me things from their intimacy. Given that, the stories, dialogues, and examples are genuine and free of any impropriety, as at the time, there was no consideration of recording anything, absolutely nothing! I want to emphasize that, based on what I heard and continue to hear from people, regarding the behavior of men and women, regardless of nationality, convictions, principles, and even religious beliefs, feelings flow, will dictates, and the rest happens. What will be, will be, and it will be with all the properties that involve sex; that is, without shame, without limits, and without fuss. In this way, even if someone comes to reprimand me regarding the content, what is said will be unsaid because I will not accept it, nor will I feel harmed by any statement made here; quite the opposite, the pleasure of presenting something that generates some controversy sets me free and motivated. I say motivated, but I digress to say that everything involving human beings, whether men or women, motivates me! Therefore, this is another work in which I am fully invested, and with it, I want to bring you sincerity in the facts, honesty with my principles, and free thought to sharpen your meditation on the theme being addressed.

*The goal of man is to be happy;*
*the goal of woman as well; because*
*a happy man makes a woman happy;*
*a happy woman makes the whole family happy!*
*Della Santa – July 15th, 2020*

# CONCEPTS, DEFINITIONS, AND RULES

*The woman you couldn't eat now,*
*if you eat it in twenty years, it will be*
*first time. So, don't be hurry.*
*Know to wait for the right moment!*
*Della Santa - June 11th, 2020*

In general, what every woman expects from a man is that he is honest and confident in what he says and that he doesn't make empty promises. If he promises, he has to fulfill it!

What every female desire is for her man to "have" her well. Because if he doesn't, there will come a day when someone else will! And there's no use in complaining; what's in the past is in the past; and if it comes back, it won't be the same as before!

Men seem like hunters when it comes to pursuing a relationship, but women are even more so. They are just more discreet!

We know there are plenty of "wolves" out there. But women also know there are many "bunnies." That's why they take good care of their men!

Some women I've met told me the following: "I want my man to always look good for others, but only for their eyes. No touching, no getting close, no groping. I prefer that others see from a distance! Something like this: seeing with their eyes but not touching; let them watch from a distance. Leave the eating part to me!"

Others have said: "Young, muscular men like we see out there are great to look at, but that's about it. For intimacy; for sex, the preference is for those considered without special attributes, the not-so-handsome ones. They are the ones who usually get the job done and are always ready and eager. The handsome ones are too full of themselves; they enjoy it too much, and that is off-putting. Not to mention that when needed, they can hardly get the job done, and the woman is left unsatisfied. An unsatisfied woman loses her mind, goes wild, becomes like a wild animal!"

As a general rule, women are like men, but with a thinking head. Men, on the other hand, have two heads, one that thinks and one that doesn't. Even worse, it's lost; stubbornly lost. So lost that it only feels good when it's naturally erect!

Something that seems illogical but happens like this is: when a woman wants to be intimate with a guy, she wants that guy. If it doesn't work with him, another guy might be able to, but she, during the act, will be thinking of him; the one she would rather be with!

Another rule here: the female chooses her male, the one she will be intimate with; the male chooses all of them. Exception: some females choose all the males, and some males choose only one female and are only interested in her!

Within this rule lies the understanding of why men and women sometimes kill over their mate. It's idiocy, a vile act, petty, unreasonable, but we know that it happens, and it's not rare! Therefore, it's understandable but not acceptable that someone considers themselves the sole owner of the other and kills in the name of possession, even worse when they claim it's for love. It's a tremendous mediocrity!

For heaven's sake, don't get involved in someone else's relationship. It could be your brother's or your sister's, even your best friend's. Dirty clothes only in time of "blackout[1]" is that washes in the neighbor's house. Any other time, you wash it at home. And if you want to know why, you'd have to take sides, and no matter which side you choose, you'll be wrong. In a relationship, both are right. No one makes mistakes alone, and the relationship doesn't deteriorate on its own. So, both are guilty. There's no way to take one side or the other. If you get involved, know that you'll be in trouble! Your sister, your brother, your friends are yours in sentiment, but the relationship belongs to them; the choice was theirs. So, they have to solve it if there are problems. This can't be outsourced. There's no way to escape this rule!

One thing that always puzzled me is the issue of jealousy. For a long time, I wondered why some, if not many, people show so much jealousy. Since I couldn't find a plausible

---

[1] This occurred in Brazil between July 2001 and February 19th, 2002, during the second term of President Fernando Henrique Cardoso, and was probably caused by a failure to plan and invest in energy generation. A difficult period for the Brazilian population involving a lack of electricity.

answer, even after reading renowned authors, I started talking to people I had some intimacy with and asked many questions. The result didn't alarm me, but over time, I arrived at my conclusions: jealousy, as experts in the field say, is an illness, a fetish, an emotional disorder, and a difficulty people have with the possibility of loss. In other words, these people don't accept losing and have a deep-seated possessive desire, making jealousy an emulation, a perversion. But in my inquiries, this time talking "normally" with people, I understood better. Jealousy, except for serious and honorable exceptions, is simply to cover up marital wrongdoings that the person doesn't always do but has in their mind and thinks that the other person does or might do. Hence the need to stop it, to cut it off at any cost, even the cost of pathological jealousy! So, my friend, be very careful with jealousy! If a jealous man hits, hurts, injures, or kills; a jealous woman is also capable of doing the same! Several women have told me that if they find out that their man is seeing someone else, they'll go out with anyone just to get revenge. What intrigued me the most was that some of them said that even without confirming if it's true or not. As simple as this, according to them: "Where there's smoke, there's fire!" In other words, for many, no investigation is needed to confirm that the fact is true. Rumors and their sources don't matter. It's sad, but for those with pathological jealousy, that's how it is! An old friend of mine used to say: "If love is blind, my dear; pathological jealousy sees even what doesn't exist!" I would say it's essential to pay attention to certain signs, that's right. The truth always comes out. And anyone who is attentive to what is theirs will never fail to see or at least notice the obvious! Acceptance is another story...

> *Everything in life depends on acceptance...*
> *But, before accepting, it is convenient*
> *to think about more or less*
> *everything!*
>
> *Della Santa – July 17th, 2020*

# TIPS AND ADVICE

*"Love is not a trap.*
*It's just our habit*
*to enter a relationship*
*without any analysis*
*of the consequences!"*

*Della Santa – June 15th, 2016*

a) I never wanted to dissuade someone that love is blind. But honestly, after the first fuck the eyes open. There, only does not see who does not want to see!

b) Don't be fooled by a woman who asks to borrow money from you. If you lend her money, you'll end up being worthless to her, unless you are facing an exceptional situation.

c) A woman who desires you initially, well, she just desires you. If it seems like there's more to it, you need to run as fast as you can. Any oversight is an open door for disappointment.

d) If it falls into your fishnet, it's fish. But be very careful with big fish and rare beauty. This type of fish is like large watermelon and appears to be sweet: you delude yourself thinking that you will eat alone! Always remembering that there are exceptions to the rules.

f) A man who needs viagra or prosthetic to fuck, urgently needs to hang up his boots. Have you ever wondered if a woman offered you a pussy made of rubber, silicone or anything like that? Said an old friend of mine in days of yore: *"Nothing replaces the meat that pissed for me!"*

g) Do not be skeptical, my dear, believe me: there is an insatiable woman! If you do not believe, may one day suffer because of this!

h) No one deserves to be imprisoned. But a donkey man with women and especially those who treat them badly, deserves a halter! Please don't be such an idiot like that!

i) Don't believe a woman who claims to like rude and unwashed men. In reality, she simply struggles to express her desires. What she really wants and enjoys is wild, passionate sex. It's up to you to discover that. Walking dirty and smelly will never make you win; at least, someone worth their cherish!

j) You must have noticed that I'm speaking bluntly here, right? Want to know why? Because I'm addressing men, and without being derogatory, men don't need airs and graces. What they need is clarity. The clearer, the better. And if the language is straightforward, all the more effective.

k) Respect women who love other women; after all, shouldn't we also respect men who love other men?

l) You need to understand that having sex is different from making love. When you love a woman and she love you too, each of you wants to give the best of yourselves to the other. I think I don't need to explain that in this type of sexual relationship, they are making love in the practice of sex, which is just a complement to the act that started with mere affection.

m) I'd like to make a parenthesis here to say that many women also like things to be passionate. However, let's agree that when you speak to a woman in that way, it gives the impression that you're talking to a man, doesn't it? Fortunately, what I'm writing here, although it involves women, is literally from men to men.

n) You can be kind to all women, and you should. But please, if you intend to take one to bed, be direct. Women love it when a man clearly shows his desire for her. If she rejects you, it's because she wasn't interested or had someone else in play.

o) Don't delude yourself into thinking that men eat women. In practice, in reality, it's the woman who "eats" the man. After all, he goes inside, and he's devoured by her devouring tool. A friend once told me in ancient times: *"Some men delude themselves into thinking they eat women. One day, he'll learn that he lived deluded."*

p) When you no longer want a woman, it's advisable to approach her and put an end to it. If it doesn't happen this way, when she finds you with another woman, she'll act as if you were her property and that you're blatantly cheating on her.

q) Don't think that you're a great stud, that you're excellent in bed. Or at least, if you think so, don't show it to her. And if she tells you that you're great, be humble and tell her that she's the one who's "great" in bed, or whatever you want to say in that sense. It's important that she understands that you're only good because of her. She's the only reason you've become so good.

r) Don't be mistaken into thinking that by declaring your love to a woman and hearing in return that she loves you, things are settled, and you're guaranteed. As certain as two plus two is not five, she will desire other men. Desire is like eyes: it has no boundaries. But pay close attention: this doesn't mean she'll cheat on you! I'm only talking about human stimulus here; just that, and not character!

s) If the woman you love wants to be with someone else, she will be, and it will be in a way that you won't even dream of. If she lets you know, be sure that she did it out of revenge. She wanted to get back at you for a possible betrayal!

t) If you think you have a "golden penis" and can have all women, know that there are women who think they have a "worthless" vagina and can let any man enter it.

u) All women are beautiful. The ones who should think a woman is ugly are other women! If a man thinks a woman is ugly, he needs to change sides. There may be women who are unkempt, without care, etc., but ugly, not at all! There's an old saying that seems very current to me and emphasizes this very well: "Every pot has its lid!" So, if you don't like her or think she's ugly, let it go; someone else will like her!

v) Be courteous to a woman, whoever she may be. Don't be arrogant, malicious, cunning, or conceited with her. If you embody any of these traits, one day she will stomp on you. Be sure of that!

w) Watch out for a woman's reactions; she's also a human being, you know!

x) In general, women tend to think that the places men go to are 'meeting places.' Make it clear to yours that you're heading to the local pub. It's where you meet up with your group of friends or just someone to have a casual chat while having a beer, and that's all that matters. If some woman shows up, she's a lone sheep or may even be your 'competition,' not hers! Of course, every rule has exceptions; I've mentioned that before. But if she doubts it, take her to the pub with you. I believe she'll only go once!

y) Always tell your woman, without insistence, that she's the only daughter-in-law your mother recognizes or would recognize. The others were good, but for you, she's the BEST! You can even say that you hit the jackpot when you found her and achieved your dreams by marrying her!

z) Your woman is the only possession you think you have, but in reality, you don't! I say this because it's an asset that you need to win over day by day. And be sure, you will never have done enough! Women are complicated and come at a cost, but without them, there's no life! Want a deeper reflection: why do you exist?

*It should be considered a transgression
subject to penalty to declare that
a woman is inferior to a man.*

*Della Santa – March 20th, 2019*

# ORIGINAL CASES OR WITHOUT FORMATTING

*It has things that happen in the life
that they are characterized
as mere chances.
It has thing that are premeditated;
those are the things that you have
to pay if you want to make
it happens, in fact!*

*January 20th, 2020 - 06:36'*

There are times in a person's life when things happen in a way that makes them feel overwhelmed by the strangeness or eccentricity, or even the complexity of the facts. Faced with this, many resorts to vent to feel relieved of the discomfort generated. And when this outburst happens, it is pure, genuine and devoid of any pretension that is not the morbid need to relieve, get rid of the failures that occurred. So, without delay, let's go to cases, not with before remembering that they were not counted so that one day they were cataloged in book; they were only counted and will be recorded here, in full, as they were absorbed by me. Oh, I was forgetting: except for the those who are still here, I will respect the definitive absence of those who have gone for the beyond. And so, I will not reveal anyone's identity; not at all! Here are the cases:

# CASE 01

Walney, at the age of 15, was the typical handsome teenager, with a robust physique, rather simple-minded, but many women of the time found him appealing. He lived in a shack on the family property, a bit separated from the main house, indicating a level of independence for those residing there. He shared the following with me:

"I was in my shack on a Wednesday night, a beautiful moon was casting its light on the earth around 9:00 PM when I noticed someone trying to enter my house. I remained calm because, at that time, the world wasn't as malicious as it is today. I thought it might even be a friend who had just arrived and wanted to pay me a visit. So, I waited. The door was merely closed, not locked, and it didn't take long for it to swing open. To my surprise, my boss's niece, who was also my guardian, walked in. She stopped near my bed, looking quite humble, and said, 'I came for you; I want you.'

Initially, I didn't understand and asked, 'What do you mean?'

She responded, 'I said I want you!' After a brief pause, she continued, 'Don't you want me?'

Still not comprehending, as there was no time to gather my thoughts, I replied, 'I don't understand! What do you want from me?'

Her response left me even more bewildered: 'I want to have sex with you! Don't you want me? Don't you desire me?'

At that moment, my mind completely scrambled. I went to another world and returned. I was already sitting on the bed, but the world was spinning so fast that I lost all sense of reality. I looked at her and saw that she was wrapped in a blanket. While I struggled not to lose my sanity, she approached me, opened the blanket, and said, 'Are you going to have sex with me, or do you want me to give myself to someone else?'

Moral of the story: When it comes to sex, it's not just men who can be assertive; when a woman wants something, she can be assertive too, and she applies pressure until she gets what she wants!

## CASE 02

I was very young when this happened: I met a girl who, at first, seemed simple, but obstinate and very correct in her way of proceeding. I liked her and I thought we could be friends. I didn't think about dating her because I thought she would never want to get involved with a "John Doe" like me. But to my surprise she began to woo me. At the time I was serving her boss and because of this, I was always going to the company where she worked. We talked a lot, and I don't even know where I got all that talk. My shyness was such that, honestly, I couldn't even see the opportunities that came to me. She was always helpful, kind, and somehow found ways to express her satisfaction in talking to me.

And she always helpful, very kind and always giving a way to demonstrate her satisfaction in talking to me.

One day I arrived at the company and she came to meet me. We talked and, at a certain moment, she told me: - Do you want to date me?

I was taken aback, took a few seconds to respond, and, under her inquiring gaze, I said, "Yes, I do!" My face was on fire. Anyone could have noticed it!

That day she set our first date. And thankfully, because I couldn't even do it! The next day, a Sunday, as we agreed, we met at the home of a lady who was her friend. We were chatting and listening to music for a whole afternoon. Rolled up to a few kisses and the promise to meet at night, which happened....

For that night I dressed very well, wearing my best clothes, wearing my only shoe and wearing my best perfume. I remember my mother asking me, "Where are you going all dressed up like that?" I said to her, "I'm meeting my girlfriend. I finally found someone to date!" My mother put her hand on her chin and stared at me, I think, thoughtfully. And now I can imagine what she thought at that moment and that it should be more or less like this: "My son is grown up, he is already dating!" I was then fifteen years old. And there I went to meet what, at that moment, was my goddess, the expected.... Young when wait a little, think that he waited a lifetime. It's funny, hahahaha! I thought, laughing internally.

That night, I also had my first disappointment with a woman: she appeared with a ring on the ring finger of her right hand, indicating she was engaged. I was devastated by that, suffered a lot, but I had already started something, so I decided to continue the relationship. Actually, I only truly understood the magnitude and consequences of my decision when the guy, who was 17 years older than me at the time, wanted to kill me. I took a big risk, but everything turned out fine. We broke up, and I was left with the disappointment of wanting someone who seemed to want me but was already committed.... I almost became a pawn in her hands, but it gave me some experience. I went out on the tangent and my life took almost normal course...

Moral of the story: Anyone who throws themselves headlong into the unknown risks getting lost. So, before entering any door, make sure there's a map to guide you. It might be a labyrinth inside. If it turns out to be one, it doesn't hurt to have an easy way out. The exit door is more important than the entrance!

## CASE 03

João Pernambuco was a strong and good-looking guy, at the time in his 40s, and I was just an 11-year-old when I met him. He always gave me some odd jobs to do, and I was pleased with these tasks because they earned me a few bucks. I needed those bucks because I was lacking in many ways, so any help that came my way was very welcome. But let's get back to the case: João Pernambuco was married to Mariinha, and they were constantly quarreling. She accused him of being a womanizer, and in my childishness, I didn't quite understand it. The fact is that they had their disagreements on a recurring basis, so much so that I got used to it. I even thought it was normal in married life, but it wasn't. I only realized this when the worst happened.

One Saturday afternoon, I was peacefully at home when Juqueta, a childhood friend, rushed in and said, "Do you know what happened? Do you know?"

I was terrified by his question because, after all, he didn't even greet me when he arrived. So, trying to remain calm, I asked him, "What happened? Is there a problem with someone in your family? Your mother?"

Without hesitation, he said, "No, man. It's about Mr. João Pernambuco. Dona Mariinha killed him!"

That news hit me like the Sputnik rocket. I jumped off the stool where I was sitting and inquired, "What? What's going on, man?" This time, he shook his head, emphasizing the words in a soft tone and said, "What you heard is true; Dona Mariinha killed him... He hit her, and she hit him on the head with an ax!"

I once heard Mr. Honório, an elderly man accustomed to old sayings, say, "Hitting a woman is like stepping on a snake's tail: you'll get bitten for sure!"

I put my head in my hands, thinking, "What now?" João Pernambuco was a strong man, capable of holding a bull by its horns; in fact, I saw him do that once during cattle loading.... And suddenly, everything that had happened up to that point was becoming a covered past overshadowed by death—the death of the main character in this story, which was not mine but his.

I arrived at João Pernambuco's house and found him lying in a casket. At that time, there were no dedicated funeral spaces, and everything happened in the deceased's home or a close relative's. I remember he was buried on the same day, and my mind didn't register anything about an investigation. As for Mariinha, she was arrested on the spot and then disappeared. I never heard about her again. The fact is that couple fights should be avoided because when it gets out of hand, the result, when it ends cheaply, is separation. However, what usually happens is the death of one or the other. Today, to a significant degree, we see that femicide represents a much larger number, thereby inflating the statistics of murders involving marital disputes. In this context, the female side is at a disadvantage, but in reality, everyone loses because the fact forces us to consider and accept an exorbitant number of permanently broken families.

Moral of the story: If you run, the nasty beast might catch you, but if you stay, the beast will devour you. So, run! If the beast catches you, at least you tried!


## CASE 04

In this specific case, I'm going to talk about privacy. When two people come together in matrimony or not, but join in some way, we say they become one. This is a beautiful concept, but it doesn't hold in practice. I'll explain why: they are not together all the time. One can share the truth of their workday with the other, but will the other truly understand that they've been told the truth? I won't dwell on these observations too much, but even with this, you can get an idea of why this concept doesn't work. It's a good principle and could indeed be the cornerstone of a marital relationship. I leave it to you, dear reader, to think about this and try to find meaning in what I've just said. To me, it's quite clear. But to me, and to you? Think about it...


The cell phone, that marvelous device initially invented by Nokia Bell Labs and later improved, can also be a nuisance in many people's lives, especially those who haven't understood how it should work. In fact, this device should be named "APUPIN" (Aparelho de Uso Próprio Intocável, meaning "Device for Personal Use, Untouchable"), not a cell phone. Perhaps people would respect individual use more if it had a name like that. But even if they just respected it, that would be good! Let's get to the case...

I arrived at a small bar where I'd go from time to time to have a beer and chat with friends who might be there. When I arrived, I was surprised to see two friends who, upon seeing me, immediately invited me to join them. I accepted. These were two young ladies, both married, and they were there chatting and having soda. At a certain moment, one of their phones rang, and as she answered, the other's phone rang too. She promptly answered. I felt a bit awkward because, as a habit, I always ask for permission and move away from people when I answer a phone call so as not to disturb them. Strangely, to me at least, they didn't do this. So, I had to overhear part of their conversations, which, in both cases, were short. At the end, one of them said, "Wrong number. Someone was insisting and wanting me to confirm that this phone belongs to someone I don't even know!" The other's case was more or less the same, but she summed it up by saying it was a mistake.

After this, we went back to our conversation as usual. At a certain point, one of them said, "I was thinking that if this call had happened on my husband's phone, I'd think he was having an affair!" The other, smiling, said, "I was thinking the same thing! What is the head of a woman, right!"

Moral of the story: You shouldn't snoop through your partner's or spouse's phone because you might end up seeing something that doesn't exist but that you think does because you found some trace of it. And I think I don't even need to say that this will have implications on your relationship, right? Therefore, my "APUPIN" is mine. Your "cell phone" is yours!

## CASE 05

Petito was a childhood friend who was quite interesting. He had a way of saying things that, even though it was meant as a joke, he sounded very serious. He got his nickname because he never grew. On the contrary, he had a big head and an exaggerated "pistol" (probably referring to a slang term for a male's private parts). To give you an idea of his size, I was considered a short guy, and he, being two years older than me, was at least 15 centimeters shorter than me. Hence, the nickname suited him.

Well, this kid was considered a dick, no shame or as you want to classify. The truth is, he sang any girl he talked to. Then there was a Nerinha who was always in the middle of the class and that Petito kept calling her with the expression: "Let's go fuck, Nerinha?" And this was happening in front of everyone. He didn't respect his mates, or his classmates, or even his mother. From time to time I found the mother fighting, calling his attention because of this mania of singing all the girls.

Some things, if not corrected in time, can turn into a tragedy. This guy grew more defiant and, even though he didn't grow in size, he became a tremendous scoundrel. One time he took an interest in a girl. She was in the early stages of adolescence, and he was almost reaching adulthood. By that time, I had lost contact with him for several years, but there were always some old acquaintances who would tell me stories about him. And so, I found out that he showed his "pistol[2]" to this girl, and her brother, when he found out, didn't like it. He confronted Petito and reprimanded him. However, in response, the troublemaker said, "I showed it to her, I'm going to sleep with her, and if you make a fuss, I'll take care of you too!" The result was the following: the guy shot him in the face, and he ended up in a seven-foot-deep hole, as people used to say back then. I was shocked to hear this, but I had no doubt that nothing good would come out of it. It reminded me of a friend who was the father of four daughters, and another friend, who had three sons, once made a quip: "Secure your mares because my colts are running free!" To this, the father of the daughters replied, "If your colts aren't 'handsy' (meaning 'queer' in this context), they should know that my fillies are in my pasture, and if a colt enters my fence, I'll welcome it with a shotgun!"

Moral of the story: Be polite and respectful. Respect what belongs to others so that they will respect what is yours! Don't talk about what belongs to others so they won't talk about what's yours! Treat others as you would like to be treated!

---

[2] Pistola is the same thing that penis. It's a slang term in Brazil.

## CASO 06

Certain day, Walney and I were selling vegetables, and while passing through a street with the name "Índio" (I found the name strange, but it was normal since the neighborhood was named Aldeia), a young woman, probably in her twenties, called us over to choose some vegetables. She ended up making a purchase, and as we were leaving, she turned to us and said, "Next time, you guys come by, and I'll buy more." We were delighted with the offer and promised to visit more often. And we did. But one day, for some reason I can't remember, I couldn't go, so Walney went alone. That day, he returned home elated, almost unable to contain himself, waiting for me to return from where I was to tell me what had happened. He said something like this: "Ge, come here, I want to tell you something." I was anxious and wanted to know right away what he was talking about, but he refused to say anything. He said, "Let's go to my house; I'll tell you there." So, we went there.

When we arrived, he made me sit on the bed (he didn't have a table with chairs or even a stool, so we would sit on the bed), and he began to speak: "Do you remember that woman from the Índio street?" I replied, "Yes, I remember. But what about her?" He went on, "I went to sell vegetables to her, and I ended up giving her a head of lettuce. You know what she did?" I was confused, not understanding much, and asked, "So, she had coffee with you?" He responded, "No, dummy. She pulled me into her house and saying so," "Come here and I'll give you a little bit of me!"

He said it with a laugh, though I'm not sure if he was laughing by her or by me.

Moral of the story: A woman seems to give in to a man for any reason, but the reality is that she gives when she wants to give. However, on that day, I understood that a head of lettuce can have a value invaluable. It all depends on the moment!

## CASE 07

Mr. Nuno was an Italian from Crotone, located in the Calabria region, who somehow ended up in my town. According to his stories, the city where he was born was founded in the 8th century BC. He didn't like to talk much about his birthplace; he was genuinely grateful to Brazil, which he regarded as the country that had welcomed him like a son.

Mr. Nuno loved fishing, and this was his favorite pastime in my town. The "Rio das Velhas" that flowed through it at the time was teeming with fish. We developed a good friendship, and we would go fishing whenever we had some free time.

Once, we went fishing on a Friday and didn't return until Sunday. Of course, his wife was informed about this fishing trip. It was so well arranged and approved that, when we left his house, his wife... (I don't remember her name, so I'll call her "Laura") even wished us well and said, "Go with God!"

We fished, had some cachaça (Mr. Nuno loved a good cachaça), and had a great time. We enjoyed ourselves and even caught a few fish, not many, but as he used to say, "The important thing is the distraction!" in his Italian-accented Portuguese.

We headed back to his house in his old but well-maintained pickup truck. Mr. Nuno was a mechanic and kept his old companion in impeccable working condition. During the journey, we made a stop in a rural area to relieve ourselves. Strangely, when you're close to the water, you don't feel the urge to urinate, but as soon as you move away, it hits. As we were doing our business, a beetle or wasp, I'm not sure which, brushed against Mr. Nuno's neck. He complained that he was stung, but I didn't see anything, just a slight redness. We continued without much concern.

An hour and a half later, we reached Mr. Nuno's house. We had to stop there first to unload our fishing gear. As soon as we arrived, I was invited inside for a glass of water, and I accepted. After entering, Mr. Nuno called Laura, and when she approached, he gave her a gentle kiss on the cheek. She seemed not to have noticed my presence, put her hands on his shoulders, and asked, "Where have you been?" He looked at her as if he hadn't understood the question. She repeated the question, and he jokingly replied, "Well, well, we went fishing. Wasn't that what we were supposed to do?" She immediately said, "What's that mark on your neck[3]?" She pointed to a now very visible red mark on Mr. Nuno's neck. He defended himself by saying it was just a bug that had brushed against him when we were on our way back home.

She, very suspicious, added, "I don't know, you men aren't trustworthy!" She expressed some doubts, and Mr. Nuno, who had appeared very peaceful until then, became exasperated. I saw the moment he put his hand into his pants' zipper, revealing a noticeably red penis, with which he smacked the edge of the table, saying, without losing his Italian accent, "Look, Laura. My pestola is the same size, same thickness; it's not smaller or thinner. Therefore, nothing happened!" She responded, "Well, that's good to know, but I still don't trust men!" They continued to argue for I don't know how long. Witnessing this, I grabbed my things, which weren't many, and left for my home. I never

---

[3] I don't know if it happens nowadays, but at that time when a man went out with a woman and she was liking the guy, gave him a blow job in the neck as if he was stamping, leaving his mark with the implicit sayings:" That man is mine!"

went back to Mr. Nuno's house. I didn't stop being his friend, but I preferred to avoid that kind of embarrassment.

Moral of the story: Your wife may say she trusts you, but if she notices something different, not necessarily a lipstick mark but anything she finds suspicious, she'll make it clear she's suspicious and won't even acknowledge the presence of a friend who is there. At least, that's what I felt at that moment, and I never forgot it!

## CASE 08

I was still a boy when this case happened...

At that time, good times, Walney and I went every Tuesday and Thursday to deliver goods to establishments in the bohemian zone. At that time this kind of place was very badly talked about, given the kind of trade regarded as immoral that was to make a living selling sex. The concubines of these infamous places, though good-looking, were not accepted by society and far from being well-regarded by the ladies who had their husbands to preserve. The 'sealed' girls, these are not even spoken: they did not pass near those labeled as harlots.

Young women who had lost their virginity were often shunned or quickly dispatched to the bohemian area, unless, of course, they were married off to a man they might not have chosen, but marriage was the immediate and acceptable solution. In those days, exceptions were rare. Sometimes, when the family had influence, a girl would be sent to a convent and would emerge years later as a nun. Other times, if the girl were considered a potential spinster due to societal expectations, she would be told that she had lost the only thing she had to offer, her honor. This was a misguided view, but that's how it was for a long time. For men, if they were found involved with the wrong women, they would either marry them, disappear, or end up in a wooden box, usually covered with lilac fabric.

Due to a delay in the delivery of goods from the countryside, the Thursday delivery was pushed to Friday. On this particular day, while making their last delivery, they encountered a scene that any teenager or pre-teen would love to see and, if it were today, even film or record a video of. The young woman from the bohemian area was seducing a man who appeared to be returning from work and had perhaps ended up there for some unknown reason. She was embracing him without giving him any chance to escape. She said, "Where's the money you have there, where is it?" He replied, "I don't have any money; I'm coming from work and haven't been paid yet." She insisted, "Yes, you do! Let's have a beer and go to my room. I'll give you a lot of love; I'll make you very happy. Come, come! Come with me!" He said, "I can't, I have to leave..." But she persisted, not giving him any time to react. At this point, she was embracing him more passionately, kissing his neck, and calling him "my dear." Her underwear was visible, revealing her shapely legs. The two boys watched in astonishment, almost paralyzed. They felt as though they were under a spell, completely absorbed in the moment.

They had never seen anything like it, so natural, captivating, and enchanting. In those days, such scenes were only found in movies, and even then, they were either prohibited for those under 21 or restricted to those over 18. There they were, captivated by this sight. The woman seemed as if she wanted to merge with the man, to become one with him.

Suddenly, a stern voice interrupted their entranced state, saying, "What are you boys doing? What do you think you're doing? Get out of here immediately! This isn't a place for you!" They quickly realized they had done something wrong. They discreetly snuck away, but not without one last look at the captivating scene. Both Walney and me appeared to move in perfect harmony, looking at the scene simultaneously. When we got home, Walney taught me how to masturbate. He said, "When you can't have sex with a woman and you're feeling frustrated, you can masturbate to relieve yourself." Then I asked him, "But isn't that a sin?" without understanding the reasoning behind it. Walney reassured him, "Of course not. They do the same to us in return!" I've found this strange but accepted it. Walney was my idol, and he knew everything when the I knew nothing. After all, Walney was four years older than me!

I kept this episode in my head for a long time. I understood and accepted that the man needed to make money if he wanted to have a woman. This was so true for me, for I saw with my own eyes that this woman was not only rubbing herself, but also looking for that man's money. I saw and heard clearly!

Moral of the story: Children take note of everything they see, and with proper guidance, they learn and shape their lives accordingly. Money can help, but it can also hinder and lead people down other paths, so it's not everything.

## CASE 09

At 19 years of age, I met Railda. She was a girl from a simple, humble family by nature and quite diversified. Fate had it that she was born a year after my mother brought me into the world. We began to date, and shortly after, I met her sister, a young lady who, at that time, had collected thirty-four springs. We had a strong bond, and she, the older sister, often sought my advice on her decisions. She demonstrated a lot of confidence in me. The relationship had progressed significantly, over a year or so. I was a young man without prospects for improving my life, just dating and not considering anything more serious, like getting into a committed relationship or marriage. How could I think of something that would require assuming all the expenses of a household without having the education or a profession that provided a decent salary? Dating was the best option, preferably without commitments.

The two sisters, Railda, my girlfriend, and Renilde, my sister-in-law, were at opposite ends of the spectrum.

Renilde was the eldest in the family, while Railda was the youngest. On one of my days off from work, as they often accompanied my movements to plan leisure outings and other activities, I was invited to have lunch at Renilde's house. As I was accustomed to this, I accepted. After lunch, we lazily lay down on some cushions placed on the carpet and started talking. After a while, Railda, feeling sleepy, went to her room, leaving Renilde and me in the living room, chatting.

At one point, Renilde said to me, "I didn't want it to be this way, but after a year of dating, it won't be long before you sleep with my sister." She paused, and I was startled. She continued, saying, "Don't be alarmed. I like you a lot, which is why I have the confidence to talk to you this way. My sister is eager to be with you." She paused again and then continued, "I just want you to do things properly. There are many men out there who don't know how to treat a woman. They think it's just about having sex, thrusting inside, give a climbed, and leaving it at that. Do it right. If you're going to do it, do it properly, use protection, try not to get my sister pregnant. Besides, be a gentleman, be good to her, don't leave her frustrated. I'm sure you'll be the first man in her life. I also know that you don't want to exploit her, but if you don't sleep with her, someone else will. She wants it." She paused once more, long enough for me to swallow hard a few times, and then continued, "You're young, you have a lot of life ahead of you, but there's no point in running away from what you want. The flesh is weak. When she opens up to you, I know you won't resist. So, I ask you again, do it properly. You might end up getting married, or even if you don't, she may marry someone else, and I don't want her to carry any trauma. In our town, there are many unhappily married women, depressed because of their relationships with their husbands. Many of these men don't know how to treat a woman in society or in bed, and such men leave us, women, extremely frustrated, lost. And many only find themselves again in the arms of someone who knows how to take care of a woman and do it properly."

From that day on, we became closer friends, and she confided in me about many things I couldn't have imagined in the female world. She gave me various tips on how to treat a woman, the care a man needs to have for his partner, the need for new actions, surprises, and affection to make her happy. She always emphasized that a happy woman would do anything her man desires. And if she isn't happy, she only acts out of obligation or even under pressure from her tormentor. At this point, she made it clear that a man who isn't good is a torment to a woman.

It was a great period, but it ended. Our friendship had become so frequent, our need to talk was so strong that even on days when I didn't meet my girlfriend, my sister-in-law would call me to chat. And so, one day, this routine led to suspicion. Suddenly, Railda believed I was having an affair with her sister and wanted to end our relationship. She didn't know that there was nothing between Renilde and me. Even though Renilde had once told me that if I weren't her sister's boyfriend, she would definitely pull me into bed. What might have pushed this belief was that, at the young age of 35 and 18 years of marriage, her husband told her that she was too old and he needed to make an exchange. Personally, on that day, I don't know if I felt more pity for her or him. I have always said, and I will say it throughout my life: you might not want a woman, but never say you don't want her because she's ugly or old. In any case, when it comes to your wife, it becomes a crime. And if it's a crime, there should be consequences! Fortunately for him, I never even considered becoming his executioner, even though he deserved it. To make it clear, Renilde and I never had anything more than our conversations and necessary confidences for both of us. The sister didn't want to believe it or chose not to accept it because she wanted something else from me, perhaps marriage because when it came to sex, with experience or no experience, I was already providing that.

After that, they moved to another city, and I never saw them again. It may have been yet another twist of fate.

Moral of the story: Everything in life is temporary. You can either seize the moment or regret not having done so. What has passed will not return, at least not in the same way or with the same intensity. It's one thing to like someone; it's another to do what is convenient for you. Life isn't always straightforward, but at that moment, it happened that way.

## CASE 10

After the episode with the engaged woman, I went through a period of not wanting to believe in the female population for a while. However, destiny plays with us, turning us into doormats, and within our needs, it sneakily blesses us with new adventures. I met Lecinda. She was a very beautiful girl, full of charm, and charming brunette girl. It was also very simple, but the kind that when I arrived in the places the boys looked, and very carefully. She then wore a lipstick grape flavor, (I came to know it later) that was just too much! Her smile looked like a prelude for a kiss....

I was invited to a wedding party and attended. I found some friends there. During that time, things were very simple. There were no special venues for this type of party, only the one club we had, which was usually expensive. As a result, family parties were typically held at home.

The buzz of the party had been going on for a while. People were dancing, chatting, and the atmosphere was joyful. Lecinda passed by, gave me a nudge, and moved on to another room. I initially stayed alone and later, two of my friends joined me. Suddenly, a very attractive girl appeared, introduced herself, and said she was ready to dance. One of my friends declined, saying he didn't know how to dance. The other one agreed, and they went to the dance floor. Two or three songs later, they returned. I commented that they had danced very little. She stepped forward and said she wanted to dance with me. "Perfectly,"

I said. I got up, offered my hand to her, and we went to the dance floor. We danced and talked, and she told me her name was Jucineide. I found it interesting and made that clear. But I realized that the conversation wasn't the type that pleased me. I limited myself to being a gentleman and waited for her to initiate us stopping. She seemed to read my thoughts and asked, "Can we stop now? I'm quite tired... You can invite me to dance again later, okay?" "Perfect," I agreed, without much enthusiasm in my voice. I thanked her, and she made a gesture like a contented lady and walked away.

Back at the table, my friends commented, "You've got it all, huh! The girl was into you!" I smiled and shrugged. I honestly didn't think she was into me. Later, at my friends' insistence, I went to invite her to dance again. To my surprise, she snubbed me, saying she didn't feel like dancing. I must have turned red, yellow, white... Back in those days, during the era of the "pé de valsa," the term used for someone who liked to dance (different from today, where they call them "forrozeiros"). But those with strong spirit, as my mother used to say, are not left unprotected. At that moment, Lecinda walked by, and to my surprise, she reached out her hand, saying, "Come and dance with me, dear, come!" Of course, I went. And we danced. During the second song, she said to me, "I saw that girl 'snob' snub you. I was angry. You don't deserve this. She's annoying and doesn't know what she's missing. Stay with me, stay!" I nearly fainted at that moment. I never imagined this could happen to me. Later, receiving all that affection and attention, with the other girl passing by and seeing us together, "in love," she made a spiteful comment that those around could hear: "Hmmm, how quickly people fall in love around here!" Upon hearing this observation, my companion replied, "We don't live in a big city, but we know how to appreciate people. We're from the countryside, but we're not fools." And that was it. Later, I found out that the girl, Jucineide, had come from Brasília-DF for the wedding. The groom was her cousin.

Moral of the story: Although it wasn't my case, the lesson here is that sometimes we look so far away when what's best for us is nearby. All we need to do is shift our attention, and we'll find it!

## CASE 11

I met Ezequiel when I was teaching a course for young adults. At that time, he was 40 years old, married, with a son who was 20 years old and a daughter who was 15. Everything seemed normal in his life. You could say that a person in his age group was in full development. And he was, except for his false wisdom, the lack of proper guidance in his upbringing.

Ezequiel received compensation that was enough for him to start a small business and buy a car that I would never buy for myself (he only bought it because his former boss had one, and he wanted the same). But his foolishness didn't stop there. He became involved with a young lady 24 years younger than him, just a year older than his youngest daughter.

Ezequiel was very reserved, and as a result, he seemed distant from people. At that time, I was often sought after to talk to those who were facing problems. It was an interesting practice: whenever someone had a problem, which was quite frequent, management would send them to talk to me. In reality, I listened more than I spoke, but when I was given the opportunity to give my opinion, I tried to do so in a practical and logical way that encouraged people to think about their actions. One day, Ezequiel asked to speak with me, and I agreed to meet with him after my class.

He began by saying, "Sir, I'm filled with problems. Could you help me?" I paused for a moment to consider what I had just heard before replying, "If I can help, I'd be happy to. Please, go ahead." He seemed to regret entering my office, but with my encouragement, he continued, "I'm filled with problems..." I replied, "Yes, you mentioned that, but what problem troubles you?" He hesitated before saying, "I don't even know where to start..." I reassured him, "Start from the beginning; that's how you should begin." I said it playfully, trying to put him at ease.

After some contemplation, he began, somewhat hesitantly, "I'm in love with a girl, and I don't know what to do... She's much younger than me." I glanced at his face and remembered that I had the profiles of all the students. It was easy to recall his age: 40. I asked, "What's the problem with being with her?" He paused, then replied, "The problem is that I'm married..." I questioned him further, "And you're married, so what? Do you have children? Have you been married for a long time?" He answered confidently, "I've been married for 21 years, and I have two children, a 20-year-old son, and a 15-year-old daughter."

I thought for a moment before asking, "So why do you think I can help you?" He responded, "I hope you can guide me on what I should do." I felt a tremendous responsibility on my shoulders after hearing this from him, so I asked, "I need to know more. I can't rush into this. What's your relationship like with your family? Do you get along? Is there any conflict, unusual conflict in a married life?" He admitted, "Yes, there is." I inquired further, "What kind of conflict is it?" He stated, "She cheated on me!" Hearing this, I asked, "When did she do that? How did it happen? And why did she do it? Can you provide any answers?" He began to explain, stating that he noticed his wife was very frigid, didn't pay attention to him, forgot almost everything, neglected her household duties, and was only concerned with the beauty salon she frequented. Their married life seemed non-existent...

At this point, I interrupted him, asking, "And where does the young girl fit into this story?" He said, "Well, I met her a little before I noticed all of this. I think my wife got jealous..." I interrupted again, saying, "Ah, and what did you do to remedy the situation?" He replied, "Nothing. I thought everything was normal, at least until the day we were alone, and the girl pushed me onto the bed... Before I knew it, I was on top of her, and we had sex." I probed, "And from what I understand, it didn't stop there, did it?" He replied, "No, not at all. From then on, we became closer and closer. We initiated a series of meetings, which happened almost every day."

As he told me the story, I couldn't help but say, "I understand. Things often happen like this." He replied, "Yes..." and that's where he left it.

This reminds me of what a friend once confided in me: "My man can be with any woman he wants. He just can't bring diseases home, can't let me go without, and can't let me find out that he's with other women!" Around the same time, another friend told me, "It's even good for a man to be with other women; he ends up being better in bed, and if he's fair, he treats his woman even better! It's just not good to be careless, a scoundrel, or an idiot to the point where the wife finds out. Anyone would feel like a fool in such a situation!" This same friend once told me, "A woman who has a good man, if she's smart, won't bother him with nonsense, won't try to be the boss, or be possessive. A foolish woman snoops around a man's things, wanting to know everything he does, monitoring him all the time; she's the one who ruins the relationship! For a man to be good, he has to be free. A man who isn't free is like a caged bird: his song is sad!" She concluded this part of her speech this way, and later, she told me many other things that I don't think are appropriate to include here.

I pondered the Ezequiel case before taking a stance, and when I did, I tried to be straightforward:

"At this point, it seems like you've made up your mind, haven't you?"

He lowered his head before replying, "No, I haven't. I want you to help me! I'm in a real mess!"

"But how can I help you? You're the one who has to make a decision. What I say won't change what you have in mind, will it?"

"Honestly, I don't know. But please, help me. I have to figure out my life!"

"Very well," I said. "To what extent are you willing to bear the consequences of your actions?"

"What do you mean?" he asked.

"It's simple," I explained, "what you'rc doing will create significant tension between you and your children. You'll have two families to support. How do you feel about that?"

"I hadn't thought about that," he admitted. "I think I got carried away in the moment..."

"Then it's time for you to think this through and try to do things more balanced. You have a family, your financial situation, and a lot to manage. Can you handle all of this without remorse and ready to face many demands? If you can, it's easy."

He thought for a moment, and I gave him time. Afterward, he said, "Give me some guidance; I'm not seeing anything clearly. I need to think about how to resolve this."

"Alright," I told him firmly. "You can't make a decision like this hastily. I'll make a small list of things for you to consider, and when you think you can organize your thoughts, come back to talk to me, okay?"

"Okay, Professor."

I then wrote down the following on a piece of paper:

01- Four families;

02- Money;

03- How to support three families;

04- Managing your psychology;

05- Taking care of everyone's health, including yours;

06- Where is the way out?

He took the paper and asked, puzzled by the words, "Four families... Can you explain, Professor? I didn't understand."

With patience, I explained each item in detail:

"Item 01 refers to her family, your wife's family, your own family, and the family you've created with your wife and children.
Item 02 is about evaluating your financial life. Whether the money you have and your expected income will be enough to cover all the expenses you'll have from now on if you decide to continue this situation. Concerning these three families, think about your wife and children, the family you're embracing now, and your car. Your car, as I mentioned, is like another family that requires maintenance. The choice is yours."

He seemed to understand, but he asked, "And what about the other two items? What do they mean?"

I replied gently but clearly, "Do you think you have the psychological strength to handle the pressure from the families involved and society? I assure you there will be a lot of pressure. And if you or someone in your life has a health issue, do you have the ability to deal with it? As for the way out, it needs to accommodate you and all the problems your actions are causing, without hurting these people. Remember that these are loved ones who have been part of your life and shouldn't be left hanging, as it would lead to your suffering much more. Think it over."

He stayed with his head down for a while, not saying anything. When he finally looked up, he was in tears. I waited for him to regain his composure and then said, "Go home. Think about everything I've told you, and when you believe you have your own answers, come talk to me again. I want to know what decision you've made, alright?"

He wiped away his tears, thanked me, and left. I stood there, lost in thought. I had seen something similar before, and in my opinion, the decision he had made wasn't the best. "I just hope this time it's different," I thought to myself.

Ezequiel disappeared for two weeks. When he reappeared, he was cheerful, with a wide smile, and immediately said, "Professor, I've decided! I'm leaving my wife and going with the other woman. I can't, I can't and don't want to live without that girl!"

Upon hearing what I just heard, I honestly felt there was nothing more to say, at least not from my side. So, I nodded, wished him good luck and success in life, and he left. He dropped out of the course midway, disappeared completely, and I didn't hear anyone mention him. Since I didn't know his family, I couldn't inquire to find out any information. But that's how life goes; time passes, as everything does, and should. After all, nothing, absolutely nothing, is indifferent to the passage of time, not even memories, whether they are good or bad. It may not change in the same way for one or the other, but one thing is certain: it changes.

Sometimes later, you'll soon find out how long, I was in Montes Claros, a city in northern Minas Gerais, on a Saturday. I used to go there from time to time, and as always, I visited an agricultural fair. I really enjoy fairs, and everywhere I go, I always check if there's one and where it's located, so I can pay a visit, even if I'm not planning to buy anything. As I was walking around, guess who I ran into? That's right, Ezequiel! When he saw me, he approached, showing some happiness and said in a friendly tone, "Professor, it's great to see you!"

I replied, "Ezequiel, my friend, how are you doing?" I noticed a hint of sadness in his eyes. But then he told me, "I'm okay, Professor, but I've lost everything. I'm trying to rebuild my life, but it's tough. This is the result of a poorly made decision. Look..." He said this and pointed in a direction. I turned to look, and just a few meters away, I saw a pregnant woman with an enormous belly that looked ready to give birth. I turned back to Ezequiel and asked, "Is that your wife?"

He replied, "Yes, that's her, the girl I told you about." I looked at her again and saw that she had aged a lot in such a short time, as had he. They both looked visually worn, and only two years had passed. I thought to myself, "How can a decision be so cruel?"

Ezequiel showed me his current mode of transportation: a rickety old bicycle. What he was selling at the fair was very different from what he used to sell in the well-established store he had left behind. All of this made me reflect more deeply on the matter: our choices shape our destiny. If we find suffering, we are the ones who seek it. This reminded me of an old and wise priest I had known. We had long conversations back then, and at one point, within the subject we were discussing, he told me, "Each one is their own god." Here, I intentionally used a lowercase "god" to convey that this god is different from the Almighty God we all know, the one who created everything, gave us life, and granted us free will to choose how to live it.

Moral of the story: The woman at home, the one you chose to be by your side, not out of obligation but by choice, is the one who will support you in perpetuating as the man everyone should be. Unless, of course, you consistently make poor choices. In that case, my friend, the problem lies with you. Blaming the system or the individuals you choose won't help. Those who are honest with themselves accept that the object of their choice is their own problem. And if it's your problem, you have to bear the consequences of your actions, of your choices. Life is like this: you can possess everything you desire, but remember that possession is not the same as being. If you don't know how to use it properly, it will slip through your fingers swiftly. Squeezing tightly won't help; it will escape between your fingers.

## CASE 12

I met Adalberto a few years ago. At the time, we developed a good friendship, and since then, whenever possible, we spent quality time discussing various subjects. One day, during a conversation about family, I noticed that he became somewhat sad when talking about his parents. He's married and a father, but I won't go into details about his wife and children because the story I'm about to tell doesn't require that.

When I noticed he was feeling down, I wanted to know why. He ended up confiding in me due to the trust we had built over time. He said, "I am the child of divorced parents, my friend..."
I looked at him, sensing the discomfort of the situation, and said, "My dear, you're not an exception."
With some bitterness, he replied, "I know, but what bothers me is that I don't know why. They never told me why they reached that point."

"Have you tried to find out?" I asked.

"Yes, I tried, but I couldn't get anything out of my father. I've never even broached the subject with my mother. I feel awkward about it, and I've always believed that women are never wrong."

I pondered for a moment before saying, "Yes, we often think our mothers are always right. They're never wrong."

"Why are you telling me this?" He asked, somewhat apprehensive.

"I believe it doesn't matter much who was right or wrong. What's more important is where things stand now. But tell me, what do you know or suspect about their situation?"

"Well, to be honest, I know absolutely nothing. When it happened, I was already married and didn't have access to everything they did. I was caught off guard, to be honest. It seemed like my father's fault. At least, he never blamed my mother."

"I see. Your father is your mirror, and that seems to torment you, doesn't it?"

"It torments me a lot! I can't understand how two people, after becoming adults with a family of their own, can separate as if they were merely dating. I just don't understand it."

"Neither do I."

We left it at that for the day, but before parting, he made me promise to think about the issue and provide some guidance on how to resolve it. So, I went home. Over the next few days, after reading extensively about couples and recalling everything he had told me, an idea started taking shape in my mind. I remembered that he often told me his father was much older than his mother, significantly so from his perspective. Furthermore, he treated her as if she were his daughter. In my view, husbands and wives should treat each other as such. Children are different. This should be made clear within the family, out of respect from the children towards their parents. If the mother speaks, the children obey, but if the sister speaks, not always! These differences start there for me. Children shouldn't be accomplices of their mother or father; they should only respect both as their parents and protectors. Also, to the best of their ability, participate in household responsibilities. As for the rest, it evolves over time, day by day.

Our next meeting didn't have a set date but occurred on a Friday morning. We chatted, exchanged pleasantries, and he asked, "So, any news?"

I replied playfully, "It depends on what you mean by news." My friends know that even when I'm joking, I'm serious.

He smiled before asking, "You know what I'm talking about."

"Yes, I know," I responded, and this time, I took the matter more seriously. "What I'm about to tell you is straightforward."

"I want to hear it," he said, appearing anxious.

"You'll hear this: what you need to tell your father is that their separation has been bothering you a lot, and you need the truth, only that, to find peace. You don't want to make a judgment; you just want to understand what led to their separation."

He looked at me for a moment before asking, "Do you think that will be enough to get a reasonable answer from him?"

"Well, if you can be more straightforward than that, please do! From what I gathered in this case, what cannot be missing is straightforwardness."

A light seemed to go on for him, and we went about our business for the day. We bid farewell at the end of it and didn't talk about the subject again.

Days later, perhaps a month and a half had passed, we were together once more. Of course, I hadn't forgotten everything we discussed, but I was waiting for him to bring it up, which he did. He said, "My friend, I did as you advised."

"And...?" I inquired.

"We talked, and I pressed him, but he didn't tell me anything. I asked if he wasn't concerned about what was going through my mind, and at one point, he told me, 'Talk to your mother, ask her the same questions you asked me. After her answers, come talk to me, and I'll tell you everything you want to know.' He concluded like that."

"And...?" I probed.

"I spoke to my mother; I put a lot of pressure on my questions, and she opened up to me."

"Did she say what you wanted to hear?"

"No. She said what I didn't want to hear."

"What do you mean? You didn't want to know the truth?"

"Yes, I wanted to, but finding out that they split up because my mother cheated on my father hurt a lot."

"Really? Is that how it happened?"

"Yes, it is."

"My father is twelve years older than my mother. When they married my mother was seventeen... It seemed normal the bond. But over time the differences were appearing. There came a time that, according to my mother, my father gave nothing in bed anymore... She, with all the fire and him with nothing. Just lay down together, but sex, absolutely none. One day she met a guy, ten years her junior, and that's where she embarked. When my father found out, they were already on a good path. My father did not accept it; I think he was right; and my mother stayed with the subject. Incidentally, he is with him to this day. But for us in the family, it was as if she knew him well after the separation!" When he had finished speaking to me, his eyes were shallow. But I noticed that he was relieved. I still asked him: "You are not sorry or hurt for having gone deep into that history?"

"No, of course not. I'll tell you everything; after all, you're like a brother to me, you've taught me many things about life, a kind of support I may never have had in my entire life. With this quest, you taught me even more. There are things we need to know, but they shouldn't become an obsession. Obsession hurts for sure!"

I understood and remained silent. Nothing more needed to be said. However, I couldn't help but recall what a friend once told me: "A woman can't blame a man for supposedly not wanting her. Perhaps the problem lies within her, not knowing how to make him stand tall or firm as he should. A lady may be talented and attractive, even young. Still, if she doesn't know how to use these qualities, any man who enters her life will be just passing through. Only the weak make their dwelling where they shouldn't."

To clarify a question that might be on your mind, dear reader: Adalberto's father, at least from our perspective, is living quite well with his current partner!

**Moral of the story:** A person can have the partner they desire, but that doesn't mean they'll have them forever. The same goes for a woman. No one owns anyone, and everything here is temporary. Make yourself appealing to someone, and you might have that person to yourself. Life's promise is continuity; the promise of individuals is pauses. But the ups and downs in the carriages of life never stop!

**Curiosity:** According to the IBGE (Brazilian Institute of Geography and Statistics), the average Brazilian man lives approximately seven years less than women. Given this, I'd like to leave you with a reflection: why do some men persist in the practice of marrying a younger woman? Are they only thinking about reproduction, or do they forget that years pass by?

*Having eclectic tastes makes you a moderate appreciator,
never an addict.*

*Appreciate what belongs to others, but give preference
to what you believe is yours. The miracle starts
at home, but only for those who have faith,
want it, and believe that something
good will happen.*

*In your home, it has to be this way,
and it will be, you just need to
believe faithfully and
do your part!*

*April 28th, 2020 – 7:59 PM*

# MANUAL FOR THE HIGHLY SUCCESSFUL MAN WITH WOMEN

*When a man realizes that he wants a woman,
he needs to do everything possible to
deserve her. And when later he
thinks he has her, he needs
to do much more
to keep her!*

*Della Santa – June 12th, 2020*

## 01- Be demanding, but don't be ridiculous!...

Being demanding means wanting to be clean, with clean clothes, well-groomed, with a tidy home, punctual, and in control of what you do. Being ridiculous is wanting all of this but not participating in any of the steps to achieve it. It's not wanting to help with household chores, not caring about the home, and thinking that the woman is the one responsible for taking care of everything. It's even worse to believe that a man's only obligation is to provide and minimally maintain the resources necessary for the family.

## 02- Be patient, but don't be a coat hanger, broom, or mop!...

Be patient with your woman; listen to her. In fact, speak less and listen more. Every woman loves a man who is available to listen to her. Many times, she doesn't even need you to say anything; she just wants to be heard. She doesn't want your opinion. And if she does, she will ask for it. When that happens, be concise, practical, and objective. Don't beat around the bush. She needs to feel your certainty when you speak. She needs to feel that you are a point of support and not someone who doesn't take a position. She needs to feel that you are the guy who is ready to support her, especially morally. Being a coat hanger, broom, or mop means not having your own opinion, letting yourself be led by her and her anxieties. So, take the time to listen and think before you speak, because when you do speak, let it be authentic, reflecting your clear opinion and your thoughts in the context of what she has raised.

**03- Be responsible, but don't act like you're all that. The man is not the backbone of the house!...**

The backbone of the house is whoever chooses to be it, whether it's the man or the woman, it doesn't matter. So, don't place yourself above it. Create an opening and allow the woman to participate in maintaining the resources. Don't force this upon her, but if she is willing to participate, accept it graciously. Men don't need to feel diminished because the woman contributes to the household finances. On the contrary, men should be happy because their woman, by contributing to the household, values everything they have even more. She knows the sacrifices involved in giving up personal money for the family's well-being. Additionally, she feels more valued and useful. So, guess what happens? You'll find a woman who's tired but profoundly grateful. Because the more a woman participates, the more valued, useful, and grateful she becomes. And grateful people are undeniably happier. In fact, a friend once told me, "Every happy woman loves to share expenses with her partner." So, men need to hear a more beautiful tune than that one, right?

## 04- Be kind to your woman! The relationship will thank you...

Kindness begets kindness. You've probably heard these many times. But do you know exactly what it means to be kind? Well, before I answer, I want to make a few considerations. It's very easy to be kind to strangers or people you don't know, those who are not part of your daily life, those who don't witness your struggles, your fatigue, your misfortunes, your raving, your work pressures, and your occasional irrationality. So why wouldn't it be much easier to be kind to the person who is by your side, the one who absorbs all of these challenges, your frustrations, and even your disappointments? Here's the answer: because at home, most of the time, you are yourself, stripped of all the pretenses of the outside world. It's at home where you're only half human, and not infrequently, the other half is an irrational animal. Now do you understand? So please, don't mistreat your woman. Be kind to her. And if you ever feel like saying or doing something impolite, go back the way you came, take a walk, take a deep breath, or just stay silent. Your relationship will thank you, and both of you,

you and her, will always be grateful. Oh, I almost forgot: being kind with words means only saying what's necessary. Know when to remain silent and have the patience to listen until your throat is sore from hearing. And being kind with gestures is about participating without machismo, with consistency. It can even mean opening the car door or pulling out her chair. It could also mean making coffee and bringing it to her in bed, even if she has never done that for you. It is not about exchange, it's about contributing. who can, must do. Those small actions encourage the other to do the same, and everyone wins.

**05- Be an opinion aggregator, not a dream destroyer!...**

Seek to understand when your woman asks you for something that might initially seem out of the budget. Have a conversation about it and try to find significance in it. Men and women often have different perspectives when it comes to household matters. Men tend to be practical, and women not always. However, there's a difference between practicality and necessity. Many times, there's something in front of us that isn't practical but is necessary. And when looked at from this perspective, with regular use, it becomes practical and normal. So, show your practical side without extinguishing your woman's dreams. After explaining in detail, if she still insists on it, give it to her! Both of you will be happy. She'll be happy because she got her desired item, and you'll be happy because you made an effort to give her what she wanted!

I always say: if you can't have everything, have what you work hard for and value it! And if you pick your woman, be aware that you've embraced the whole package. In other words, she comes with everything good and bad because all of us have both sides. Is there anyone who only has one? I doubt it! In fact, I affirm it!

## 06- Be pessimistic when something starts badly...

Many couples torment each other so much that when they're in a moment of peace, it's only a moment. It doesn't last, and it seems like they miss fighting. So, they quickly get into arguments, looking for a way to start a new fight. My dear, when that happens, run away, make a quick exit, but get out. Don't start a fight with your woman or get into conflicts with her. This wears down the relationship, weakens the marriage, and can lead to its demise. You might say that your woman won't accept you leaving, but leave anyway. Find a friend, someone you trust, to chat with, clear your mind, and get a different perspective, which could prevent the temporary chaos that would otherwise put the couple in checkmate! If you have no one available, go to church, seek refuge for the moment. Later, she will thank you. And if she doesn't, it's no big deal; it's just pride. Deep down, she's grateful. I've seen many things start well and end badly. If that's the case, something that starts poorly is more likely to end poorly. I don't think it's advisable to wait and see!

## 07- Be the one who speaks, but be careful in expressing yourself! Women only like to play games in bed...

When you're talking to any woman, be clear about what you want from her at that moment. It might even be your woman. Don't think she's entirely different from others just because she chose you. The differences end where she thinks she has you, and you have her. As for the rest, it's all the same! None of them like beating around the bush; in fact, they are very smart. When you think you're beating around the bush, she's doing the same to you and waiting to see where it leads. This is if you've piqued her curiosity. If not, whether politely or not, it depends on your perspective, she will distance herself from you. So, if you see a woman, like her, and decide to approach her, be polite, but be direct and straightforward. Women appreciate men who are decisive upfront. Later, they decide whether they want to make the decision or let themselves be led. In both cases, the man is just a pawn, unless he's not interested in her. And if everything goes well, in bed, she wants games, at least until the right moment, the 'moment of truth.' Then you can be sure she will ask, even beg, and that's when you'll see if the wait was worth it!

**08- Be conscious: size doesn't matter; it's just a detail...**

I often hear someone saying they have a small penis, and many have even told me that your woman or other women have complained about it. They complain without offense, just expressing their desire for the guy's penis to be bigger. Well, for those in the category of having a small penis, here's some advice: be caring! If you're attentive to your partner, she won't even think about your small penis. After all, during intimate moments, the primary source of pleasure for a woman is the clitoris. That's exactly where you should focus your efforts if you want to please your beloved. It's important that you do well. So, forget the small detail and concentrate on what's important: caring, which is an action in itself to set the stage. Everything will head in the right direction, and she will be happy. And if she radiates happiness, you'll be even happier!

## 09- Be a man of class: an invitation stimulates the event...

You've probably invited your woman out several times, and you've seen the positive effect it has; it's like a light turning on, and she becomes more affectionate and happy. Now I ask you: have you ever invited your woman to a motel? If you haven't, there's still time, and it's an action that can even save a marriage or any romantic relationship. When you invite your woman to an experience like that, even if she's suspicious and finds it strange, tell her that you'd like to make love in a different way, in a different place with a touch of eroticism and possible fantasies. Make it clear that it's a fantasy you have. I bet she'll like it so much that, from then on, don't be surprised if she invites you to a motel from time to time. And you'll see that, at home, the relationship will improve significantly; just enjoy and have fun!

## 10- Be a support: treat her child well...

Generally, women tend to believe that the child is theirs. In your case, you were just a tool, a part of human creation! In fact, except for rare exceptions, women tend to think they own the children they gave birth to. Also, it's not uncommon for some men to believe they own the offspring they've contributed to. Perhaps this is why Della Santa wrote in 'Learning from Life': "There is something sublime in life called parenthood. But, when facing it, remember something very important: nobody owns the child they call their own!"

And just to emphasize, my mother used to say, "I'm sure that my daughters' children are my grandchildren, but I have doubts about my sons' children!" Don't worry; there's no need to be upset because of this. My mother just meant that she didn't need a DNA test to prove that her daughters' children were her grandchildren, but she might need one for her sons' children if she had doubts! My mother wasn't literate, but she had astonishing wisdom. She was wise!

So, my friend, it's fair and necessary to treat her child well, whether the child is yours or not. Only by doing so will you have everything from her, including what pleases the man and satisfies the woman when used properly. To add a little more: a man who satisfies his woman is in an advantageous position. All women appreciate this quality!

## 11- Be surprising... Every woman loves to be surprised!

You might be great in bed, but it's pointless to keep doing the same thing every time. If a man likes innovation, fantasizes, and craves something new, so does a woman! Therefore, it makes perfect sense to surprise her from time to time with something unexpected. Forget about your own pleasure and focus solely on hers. Let her explore herself, do whatever she wants to her own body, and make her happy! If you think it's difficult, start with a good conversation. Every woman enjoys a good conversation. Talk about things she likes or encourage her to talk about herself, how she feels about any situation, and everything related to being a woman. Show interest in what she did during the day or on any other day you didn't seem interested in. From there, you'll see things flowing and can build a strong connection in bed. But please, don't just think about the bedroom; make love to her anywhere. Do it on the couch, on the table, by the laundry machine, on the bathroom sink, in the laundry area. Everything is fair game. It's even okay to take her to the wild outdoors. Women love adventures, especially when it comes to making love. If they get excited, it can happen anywhere, more so than with men. Pay attention: they're not perverted; they enjoy exciting adventures! And, as always, it's important to note that there's no rule without exceptions. I'm speaking generally, but based on what I've heard from women themselves, and I've heard from quite a significant number of them!

## 12- Be calm, but understand this: when one doesn't want to, two will argue...

Whether you like it or not, every woman has the power and the capacity to make decisions. She might not want to act, leave it to the man, be feminine, and agree to please her man. However, if she has to decide, she will do so with brilliance! As Erasmo Carlos[4] said in the song "Mulher (Sexo frágil)," but what an absurd lie!

You see, when you want one thing, and the woman wants another, unless you are 200% right, don't argue. She will find a way to be right. And then, my friend, there will be an argument if you insist, because what you want is what you want, not what she wants. Surely, later, she will apologize, but at that moment, she thought she was right. A woman will never stop fighting for what she believes in. Be happy about this because, if she believes in you, she will fight for you against the entire world if necessary! But be careful: don't be neglectful or frivolous. If you act that way, even if you don't want to argue, you'll end up in one fight, right!

---

[4] *"Erasmo Carlos was a Brazilian rock singer and songwriter born in June 1941 and died in November 2022."*

## 13- Be discreet and considerate, but remember: other women aren't better than your own...

Pay attention to one thing: never speak ill of your wife in front of anyone; if you have to talk, choose who you speak to, and preferably do it without her present. You must have seen someone speak poorly of their wife near you or with you. I'm sure you felt uncomfortable. It's true; we don't feel comfortable in such situations. The reason is simple, for many people, what belongs to others is better than what's theirs. But the truth is, things aren't necessarily that way. You're not living with them, so you don't know the true extent of their situation. Another thing, my dear: if a friend's wife compliments you, it's dangerous. Your wife will be on high alert. But if your wife starts complimenting another woman's husband, that's double trouble. You need to be extra cautious then! I'll repeat many times that every rule has exceptions. Fortunately, what truly makes life wonderful are the sincere and honorable exceptions.

Another equally serious matter, my friend, is your neighbor. The day you discover that she's attractive, don't flatter or pay attention to her. Here's my warning: your wife already noticed long before you did and she's considering putting up barriers to your eyes. Women always think that if the neighbor is attractive, their husband will desire her and they won't be able to resist. After all, you are her man, the one she chose, and the other woman will try to steal. So, you know what's best? Pretend you didn't notice, didn't perceive, and don't know anyone; even though for sharp eyes, there are no barriers that prevent them from seeing, especially when it comes to what's considered good!

## 14- Be an intelligent man with intelligence...

Every man wants to have an intelligent woman by his side and is happy when that happens. But it's no different for women; they appreciate intelligence too! Remember that, for both cases, there are exceptions to every rule. You might be wondering what it means to be an intelligent man with intelligence, right? Well, that's what I'm going to explain in this section, and I encourage you to follow along to the end.

You've likely seen people boast about their child's intelligence, their grandchild's intelligence, or even claim themselves to be intelligent. When someone says their child or grandchild is intelligent, they usually refer to a young person who can use a smartphone or handle technology, for example. This is just an example of how people often define intelligence, which, in my opinion, is far from what it truly means. Intelligence, to me, means more than just having the ability to interact with the things you see in front of you with ease; it's about managing one's life successfully. I've often emphasized that a person's life is like a business; if it's poorly managed, it can go bankrupt. And let's be clear, a child who is called intelligent usually just has an aptitude for learning or dealing with things they encounter without any real commitments; nothing more. True intelligence is demonstrated throughout a person's life through their achievements or failures. So, you can only determine if a person is truly intelligent or not after several years of life experience. Before that, it's difficult to tell. But let's get back to our focus...

An intelligent man knows not to discuss relationship issues during a heated moment. At that moment, the atmosphere doesn't allow for a productive conversation and often provokes verbal or physical aggression. He knows how to give a woman a thoughtful gift. Never give her something she'd buy for herself. Don't gift her something you'd give to your mother. Remember, you're gifting the woman you're in a relationship with, not the one who raised you. It may sound strange, but both of these women look at you differently and have completely distinct feelings towards you. Thus, they are different in relation to you, and, of course, you need to be consistent in your treatment of them. This includes gift-giving. Avoid giving the same gift to different women. If one finds out, she'll feel compared to the other, and no woman likes being compared to her rival, as all women are rivals in one way or another. If a woman claims to enjoy being compared, stay away from her; she might be a sadist!

An intelligent man doesn't think of women as sexual objects. Before his own pleasure, he thinks about a woman's pleasure and the other elements that lead up to it, taking everything into account.

To emphasize, I've heard many men say that if a woman doesn't agree with them or doesn't meet their expectations, they'll replace her. That sounds great, right? But here's a question: until when? There comes a point where this becomes unfeasible, and the one who constantly replaces others will find themselves replaced. So, based on this principle, be intelligent and change while there's still time. Once it's too late, there's no turning back. Suffering will have taken hold, become sovereign, and will take charge.

There's a special woman, the one you chose without any external influence, to be your partner, your love, your soulmate, or any other adjective you'd like to use. The important thing is that if you ever need it, she'll take care of you, out of gratitude for the good care you've given her throughout your life together.

## 15- Be a good man, but don't be a punching bag...

When I talk to mature men, those who are typically between 40 and 80 years old, I often encounter a stream of complaints and grievances. They frequently say they can't bear their wives anymore. And within these complaints, I notice a lack of communication between them throughout their lives. Now that most of them are retired, with not much to do, they don't know how to stay at home either. An idle mind is like a storage room: you pile everything up there, especially what's no good. That's when a man begins to notice things he didn't have the time or inclination to see before. He starts thinking that his wife isn't taking as good care of the house, his things, or their children, if they have any, among other things.

After a bit more time, not much, maybe a little longer, since retirement works this way: you impatiently wait for it to arrive, and once it does, there's a lot of excitement. But in six months, or you could stretch it to a bit longer, you've done everything you wanted... That's when reality sets in: now what? Now, my dear, if you didn't plan for this, if you don't have a strategy, something else to occupy your time, you'll get stressed, feel bad, and worse, you might even fall into depression. But the stumbling blocks don't end there. You start doing things you didn't do before, such as excessive alcohol consumption, gambling, drugs, and chasing after younger women. Oh, if you think I've said too much, it's because you probably haven't reached this stage yet, or if you have, you prepared for it carefully. In that case, kudos to you! But don't be fooled, as new problems emerge. Everyone believes that once you're retired, you should stop running around, stop working as if the world still depended solely on you. But that's not the case. You need to keep working to remain active and not become stagnant. There are other issues too, things I've heard a lot, from many, and I can't avoid mentioning: "When I go out with my wife, she gives me orders all the time. It's as if I'm a child and don't know how to do things!" one said. "I'm going on a family outing, and everyone wants to boss me around. It's like I got old and I'm good for nothing!" another told me. "Behind the wheel of my car, my wife tells me what to do all the time. It's as if she knows how to drive better than me!" Yet another told me: "I don't even like going out with my wife anymore because after retiring, it's like I've aged even further. I waited so long for freedom, but I can't even have a beer or a couple of drinks!" These are just a few of the many testimonies I've received, and I still get them today. I'm all ears, I'm the pastor, the apprentice psychologist, the ever-willing confidant for those who want to talk. Want to know my advice? Well, I'll give it to you: be patient, be merciful, and all related adjectives. You can't shirk your responsibilities. The person who is now bombarding you with complaints would have done so before if you had time. You did have time, but you were spared because of your dedication as a good professional, a diligent breadwinner for the family, the friendly shoulder to lean on, even when you were exhausted. You were the man who came home with a grim face because the boss had gotten on your nerves, but you were also a source of support, the gentleman you used to be. But now that time is over. Everything has an end, everything fades, everything concludes, with a period. Life is a constant process of adaptation. This starts from the moment you are born, and to top it off, we all age a bit each day, 24 hours a day, seven days a week, 30 days a month, and 365 days a year, except in leap years. Here's another piece of advice: be fair. Always be open to learning something new. Strive to do things you've never done before, even if you lack enthusiasm. Don't hold grudges. Grudges only lead to more grudges, and, in the end, everyone gets hurt! Your wife nags you because now she only has you, and her life experience, everything she's seen in her life, leads her to think that if she doesn't take care of you, you won't last. So, she's extra careful. She hopes you'll be eternal, even though she knows that everything eventually comes to an end, including life itself!

## 16- Be playful, but accept that women have the right to be playful too...

In the past, there were hardly any paved streets in my town, and tall fences were unheard of. Most yards were enclosed by a simple barbed wire fence, merely for demarcation and to keep out animals. Well, I was walking down a street when suddenly a young woman came out of one of the houses. These were simple homes, and she, wearing a full, patterned skirt, was moving her hands back and forth, swaying her skirt in rhythm, all the while singing, "My xuranha[5] woke up on fire, fire, fire![6]" I was mesmerized, watching her. When she noticed me and felt my gaze, she looked back at me. To my surprise, she was a friend from my adolescence; we had even studied together in the same elementary school class.

She stopped her movements and her singing, greeted me, and invited me inside for coffee. I accepted, and as she set the table for coffee, we talked.

---

[5] Expression that was widely used in Brazil between the 1970s and 1980s to designate, without fanfare, the pussy, the vagina, or as you want to express!

[6] Translation of the music "Pegando fogo" (Francisco Mattoso - José Maria de Abreu) – Recorded in 1982 by Gal Costa - Brazilian singer.

"You disappeared, my friend. Are you not living here anymore?"

"I'm still here. I never moved..."

"Interesting. Some people think you don't live here anymore..."

"I don't know why that is, but I never intended to move..."

"It happens. Sometimes people disappear for a bit, and those who are used to seeing them start to feel like they don't live here anymore."

"Certainly." – I nodded.

We had been talking for a while when she asked me:

"You must have found it strange to see me and hear me sing like that, right?"

I smiled at her before saying:

"I confess that I did, but when I saw that it was you, I felt reassured. You're a unique woman..."

"Thank you!"

"You're welcome! I know you well enough to know how special you are!"

She smiled before saying:

"I woke up very cheerful, and I just wanted to make fun of the song "Pegando Fogo", which I don't even know who recorded. But I sang it exclusively for myself! I didn't think anyone would be listening..."

"Hmm, I understand. And it was quite funny!" – I added sincerely. – "I believe it was more due to the excitement of this beautiful morning, right?"

"I admit that I'm a very playful woman, but I'm not the only one. There are many others out there, even if they're not always open about it, but they exist!"

"I think it's natural, although I was raised in a way that doesn't allow for that kind of thing."

"That's why many of us don't openly embrace "being playful," even if it comes naturally. However, there are others who are more open, like the singer Clemilda[7] with her songs with double meanings in the lyrics: "The Owl and the Bacurau," "Eno's Ring," "Hold on to Tadeu." She's something else! Hahaha!" – She emphasized the comparison with a hearty laugh.

At that moment, I remembered a lady I had known in my adolescence: Matilde, married and a mother of six, who was very much in tune with the present day. She always surprised the men. One day, she came up to me in her living room and said, "Want to see my panties?" And she lifted her skirt, but she wasn't wearing any... So, I only saw a very hairy private part! I was quite embarrassed at the time, but I quickly understood and learned that she was like that! A bit crazy, or maybe even entirely insane...

---

[7] Cremilda Ferreira da Silva (Clemilda) from the Northeast of São José da Laje, Alagoas, Brazil, lived from September 1, 1936 to November 26, 2014 and gave us several double meaning compositions in a career that lasted 50 years, according to Wikipedia - Free Encyclopedia.

My friend and I talked for a while about everyday topics before saying goodbye. That day, I went home with one certainty: if there are playful men, and there are plenty, there are also many women who are just as playful, and we need to accept them as they are! This is the role of a man who wants to have a good relationship with the female gender!

## 17- Be open-minded, and above all, let your love flow...

The woman, especially the enlightened, likes a man decided! So, when you're meet a woman like that, be prepared to have her, even be for a short time. Want to know how? Well, if you've shown that you're sincere, the first chance you get to hug her, let her feel your masculinity, your "pistol," why not? If she's also interested in you, she'll naturally find a way to get a little closer, a subtle demonstration that she felt and liked it. Feeling in the soul is good, but the consent of the body is crucial to show the man that he's on the right path. What the body feels and the soul consents to has a lot to look forward to! Both men and women are only slaves to the feelings they don't show. By showing what they feel, they liberate themselves, become freer, and are unquestionably ready to truly love!

## 18- Be good-humored, but if you're in a bad mood, don't be rude!

Women often complain about a man's lack of finesse in dealing with seemingly ordinary situations. They say they ask simple questions, engage in conversations with a purpose to just talk. However, men often respond as if women are trying to exploit them, taking away the best in their lives. Please, be adaptable. Don't let impulsivity get the best of you. Analyze, act with a cool temperament, be calm and confident. No one loses by being this way; on the contrary, with good women, you only gain!

## 19- Be attentive, but be mindful of a woman's actions.

When a woman asks you to do something she can do herself, do it. If she asks you a second time, do it. And if she asks you a third time, do it again. If she's a good woman and was merely testing you, you won't need to do it anymore; she'll do it herself. But if she's cunning and was testing to take advantage of your goodwill, she'll continue wanting to use you. In that case, you'll need to have a feeling to recognize her ploy and jump ship. Those who seek participation deserve it; those who want to leech should go find teats for that. Real men have principles!

## 20- Be demanding with your child, but educate you for the life. This it charms any woman that observing you!

Usually, when a man has a child, both father and child hope the child will be just like the father. Like this: like father, like son. I think that's great, but demand the following from your child: to be like you, first and foremost, they need to respect women; and secondly, respect people as a whole. And if you have a daughter instead, tell her she needs to learn to respect men. Only then will men return respect to her. Life teaches us that those who respect deserve respect, regardless of gender. This is a rule for everyone. Those who break it will carry the weight of disappointment.

## 21- Be a visionary when it comes to women.

When you see a woman in any setting and like what you see, think right away that she can be yours. Just approach her and, with skill, win her over by expressing your intentions. If you find it challenging, remember this: you already have a "no" if you don't try, but you might receive a "yes" if you do. So, what are you waiting for, my friend? Go for it! What falls into your lap easily might seem less valuable, but what you fought for, that's what truly matters. You and anyone who witnessed your struggle knows it, knows your worth! When a woman goes somewhere alone to have fun and unwind, that's all it is. But if she meets a man who piques her interest, her initial thoughts are quickly discarded.

*Seek to conquer to have and call your own. You'll only suffer if you persist in taking what belongs to others. If you've conquered it, it's yours!*

*Della Santa – July 8th, 2020*

# HEALTH CARE

*The intelligent man looks inside of people,*
*and he dresses of them to meet himself,*
*and admit himself as a work sublime*
*built up by God. However, it is*
*necessary to understand that*
*no one is immortal!*

*Della Santa – July 6th, 2020*

In the past, when someone talked about health, I didn't pay much attention to it. I can't even say it was because I didn't care; the truth is, it was a cultural lapse, a lack of knowledge. Now, after navigating the intricacies of medicine, consulting various professionals in the field, and reading literary works in this context, I feel obligated to share some of what I've learned. Forgive me for using the expression "a little," but the complexity in this field is so vast that speaking at length is best left to the professionals who initially spent six years of their lives studying the facets of health, continuing to study, research, and, undoubtedly, never stop there. After all, life doesn't stand still, and the need for new discoveries never ceases. Thus, it's a field where everything evolves, grows, and tends towards infinity.

I'm not a doctor, and that should be clear. I'm just an ordinary person with perhaps a bit more knowledge than those who know nothing or very little. So, what I'm going to discuss in this context is just speculation, not medical advice. In fact, to make it even clearer, I want to emphasize the following: what precedes a speculation is the word "give." You don't sell a speculation; you "give a speculation." If you were selling it, it wouldn't be speculation; it might even be a consultation.

What life has shown me is that men are less inclined to seek out medical attention. Many even boast about never having gone to a medical professional voluntarily. It's worth knowing that not only practice but also facts have demonstrated that everything goes well until the age of 40; after that, the decline begins. So, why not pay attention to your health before that? Diligence, routine self-care, is the best medicine because those who practice it are acting preventively. It's not about searching for diseases, as many people think, but avoiding the progression of a condition that might be in its early stages. Then, it's much easier to find the right treatment and cure. A doctor is pleased when someone consults them for preventive care but saddened when someone arrives falling apart due to neglect. In other words, a good doctor wants you to be well, making your visits to their office feel like a pleasant routine or even a stroll.

I remember that once a friend told me, after undergoing a lengthy and ultimately palliative treatment that filled his life with restrictions, "We only value our health after it's taken from us, and by then, as in my case, it's too late!"

So far, I've talked about a lot of things without being concise. Let's move on to the most important aspects, the ones that really matter: how is your health? Are you someone who takes good care of yourself? In the following steps I will list a script to guide you in a simple way in what we need for you to take better care of what needs to be the focus of our interest: male health!

# 01- PHYSICAL ACTIVITY

It's advisable to have some physical activity in your routine (it can be a walk) and engage in it 4 to 5 times a week, at least 30 minutes a day, which equals 120 to 150 minutes per week. Put idleness aside and don't wait for your doctor to tell you to engage in some activity to keep your body active. Oh, and no making excuses like "I walk a lot at work during my working hours. I don't need extra activity!" Please, push aside that thought. At work, you're working; therefore, your mind is focused on your job, not on an activity meant specifically for your body. The timing doesn't matter, but make time for it. Whether it's a gym, swimming, dancing, gymnastics, or group sports, your body will respond well, even in sexual activity, and that's crucial in a marital relationship!

# 02- INTELLECTUAL ACTIVITY

Engage in reading. Reading stimulates the brain. With a stimulated brain, it becomes easier to take care of your body because it responds more effectively to any activities you undertake to maintain physical vitality. With your mind and body consistently stimulated, your sexual side, your tool will not fail!

Within intellectual activity, you can also enjoy activities such as crosswords, word searches, playing dominoes, video games, billiards, chess, playing cards, and more. But beware: do these activities for leisure only. If they turn into vices, forget about them. Set them aside. An addiction distorts the purpose, turning something good into a game of chance with losses, not gains. In other words, what you gain intellectually, you may lose morally!

# 03- WHERE TO START

No one can do for you what is personal and depends solely on you. So, for everything I've discussed so far and what I'll discuss from here on, if you don't want to do it, no one else can do it for you. Unfortunately, you can't outsource your healthcare, physical activity, body care, and mental well-being. This is something only you can do! So, put on a brave face against reluctance, open up to the need, and take action! Go in search of what you need. Your satisfaction in the medium and long term will thank you!

## 04- ANDROPAUSE

Andropause, a condition recognized in medicine for quite some time, is an age-related decline in male hormones, particularly testosterone. Typically, testosterone, the primary driver of male sexual desire, can gradually decline after the age of 40, though this doesn't happen to everyone in that age range. Above the age of 50, symptoms associated with andropause may begin to appear. These symptoms include a decrease in libido, depression, and disinterest in sexual activity. Other tangible symptoms may include bone density loss, and the low level of testosterone can endanger cardiovascular health, among other issues. In this case, it's crucial to seek support from family, close friends, and find ways to manage stress. Physical exercise will help your body produce endorphins, increasing your mood and keeping your bones and muscles strong and healthy. Seek nutritional guidance to adjust your diet. A diet aiming to avoid excessive fat consumption but with plenty of fiber and protein is necessary to stimulate hormone production. A diet rich in minerals helps maintain healthy testosterone levels. Don't consume excessive alcoholic beverages as they tend to lower testosterone levels. Consult your doctor to maintain healthy blood circulation, which ensures your "pistol" will function when needed. Nowadays, with **Hormone Replacement Therapy** for men, it's increasingly easier to manage these symptoms and prevent their severity. Don't hesitate: consult a doctor to determine if hormone replacement is necessary if you experience the symptoms mentioned earlier.

# 05- PROSTATE

I'll start this section by saying something that left me astounded when I heard it. But there's one thing we must never, under any circumstances, avoid, and that is reality: "90% of men will experience prostate problems in their lifetime if they do nothing to prevent it."

However, it's known that the first signs of prostate changes are noticed around the age of 40. At this stage, you might begin to experience the need to urinate more frequently during the day and at night. What to do? Well, see a doctor. Medical guidance is key. The sooner you do it, the less suffering you'll endure. For an enlarged prostate, you need to consume nutrients that allow it to function normally. But here's a piece of advice: don't use miracle formulas without consulting your doctor first. They have the authority to guide you in the best and necessary way! Furthermore, don't shy away from the "digital rectal exam." It won't hurt anyone; at most, it might invade your little hole without causing harm. In reality, this is much better than an invasive surgery. Nothing can replace an original part removed from our body.

# 06- REGULAR OR ROUTINE CHECK-UPS

I will list some routine tests that your doctor will typically recommend. Of course, they know which tests are required, but it's helpful for you to have some information to avoid wasting time and poorly phrased questions, or even forgetting that you need the information. Don't beat yourself up for not knowing or forgetting to ask your doctor. The truth is, we get nervous, and that can lead to a slip of the mind. But let's move on to the exams.

## Fasting Blood Sugar:

This test measures the level of glucose (sugar) in your blood and is done after an 8 to 10-hour fasting period without food or drinks, except water. It's used to detect and monitor conditions like hypoglycemia, hyperglycemia, and, of course, diabetes.

## Hemogram:

Used to diagnose disorders like anemia, autoimmune diseases, and leukemia. The test measures levels of red blood cells (erythrocytes), white blood cells (leukocytes), and platelets.

## Urea and Creatinine:

Primarily used to assess kidney function. However, they are now most useful for chronic kidney patients, as creatinine testing is aimed at diagnosing advanced kidney problems. Nevertheless, it's essential for monitoring overall kidney functions.

## Uric Acid:

Used to evaluate the levels of this substance in the blood. Uric acid is a byproduct of purines, compounds found in the body's cells, including DNA. Excess uric acid in the blood can lead to gout or kidney stone formation and, in more severe cases, kidney failure.

## Total Cholesterol and Fractions (HDL, LDL, and VLDL):

Mainly used to calculate the risk of artery blockage and cardiovascular diseases due to cholesterol. If LDL levels in the blood are high.

## Triglycerides:

Used to check if triglyceride levels are within a healthy range as part of a cholesterol test (also called a lipid profile), which is a simple blood test. If you have any doubts about your health, don't hesitate to consult a doctor. Professional guidance is essential to prevent the worsening of any type of illness.

## TGO/AST and TGP/ALT:

Sensitive indicators of liver damage in various diseases. However, it should be emphasized that having higher than normal levels of these enzymes does not necessarily indicate an established liver disease. These levels can indicate a problem or not. The interpretation of elevated TGO and TGP levels depends on the overall clinical picture and is best determined by experienced hepatologists.

## TSH and Free T4:

Hypothyroidism is a condition caused by low thyroid hormone production. Hyperthyroidism, on the other hand, is a condition caused by excessive thyroid hormone production.

## Alkaline Phosphatase:

Used to measure levels of this enzyme in the blood. When altered, it indicates possible liver damage. Alkaline phosphatase is also found in the liver, where it's present on the edges of the cells that combine to form bile ducts -

small tubes that drain bile from the liver into the intestines, where it's needed for fat digestion.

## Gamma-Glutamyltransferase (GGT):

Used to measure the levels of this enzyme in the blood and assess liver damage. GGT is present in the cells of the bile ducts, and damage to these cells causes an increase in GGT enzymes in the blood.

## C-Reactive Protein (CRP):

C-Reactive Protein (CRP) is a protein produced by the liver, and its blood concentration increases significantly when there are signs of inflammatory or infectious processes. The level of this protein is measured through a standard blood test, aiming to evaluate the possibility of infection, inflammation, the risk of cardiovascular diseases, neoplasms, rheumatic diseases, traumas, and other severe conditions. Although the test does not indicate the specific site of inflammation or infection, an increase in its values, which is not always a cause for concern, requires evaluation by a doctor within the context of each patient to determine the relevance and whether further investigation is necessary. Additionally, when the body is dealing with an inflammatory process, the blood test can also indicate an increase in white blood cells, which are the body's defense cells.

## Urine Test:

The urine test, also known as a "Urinalysis" or "EAS (Elements Anormais do Sedimento)" in some countries, is an examination commonly requested by doctors to identify changes in the urinary and renal system. It should ideally be performed by analyzing the first urine of the day, as this morning urine is more concentrated due to time.

## Stool Test:

This test is used to look for cysts or eggs of parasites and is helpful in identifying intestinal worms. In this case, do not use laxatives or suppositories before collecting the stool, and the specimen should be refrigerated.

## PSA (Prostate-Specific Antigen) Free/Total:

Used to detect various prostate issues, ranging from benign prostatic hyperplasia or prostatitis to, in rare cases, suspicion of prostate cancer. This test is requested at the beginning of your doctor's investigations. Other tests, such as the digital rectal exam, may be included for diagnostic complementation if necessary.

## Colonoscopy:

In general, this examination evaluates the mucosa of the colon, primarily indicated to identify the presence of polyps, colorectal cancer, or other types of intestinal alterations, such as colitis, varices, or diverticular disease. It is recommended for all individuals over the age of 50.

## Important note:

When you go through your doctor in consultation, make sure you haven't forgotten anything in terms of questions or tests. Remember that you are not his only patient and that because of this he may forget some detail. Report the facts without omission. Be true! If possible, make a list of everything you need to ask. Your health thanks!

# 07- TO MAINTAIN GOOD ORAL HEALTH

It's important to take specific care of your mouth, as it plays a crucial role in your overall health. The mouth is the largest cavity in the body that directly contacts the environment, making it one of the primary entry points for harmful microorganisms. Scientific studies have confirmed that oral health is closely related to overall health, and poor oral hygiene can lead to cardiovascular diseases, diabetes, and more.

To keep your smile beautiful and healthy, you need to take certain precautions, including:

Brush your teeth daily after each meal and before bedtime, using dental floss to clean between all teeth.

Monitor your diet, controlling the intake of sugary foods, especially between meals.

Use mouthwash to maintain fresh breath and eliminate bacteria.

If you appreciate a clean and well-maintained mouth, remember that it's the same for the female population. Do your best, and you will be considered the best!

## The most common oral problems include:

## Cavities:

These are mainly caused by inadequate hygiene, consumption of sweets and carbohydrates, or complications from other diseases that reduce saliva in the mouth.

## Bad breath:

Several causes can lead to bad breath, including inadequate oral hygiene, gingivitis, the consumption of foods like garlic or onions, tobacco and alcoholic products, dry mouth, systemic diseases like cancer and diabetes, and liver and kidney issues. Prolonged fasting and sinusitis can also lead to bad breath.

## Gingivitis:

An inflammation of the gums caused by the bacterial plaque.

## Bacterial plaque:

A collection of bacteria that mainly adheres to difficult-to-clean areas, typically between the gums and teeth or on the back teeth, causing cavities and tartar formation.

## Tartar:

The hardening of bacterial plaque on the surface of the teeth.

To avoid these problems and have control over them, make sure to visit your dentist at least once a year, or according to the frequency recommended by your dentist.

# 08- EYE CARE

Eye health is one of the most critical aspects of the human body. Vision is undeniably essential for various activities we engage in daily. However, in your daily life, you may not realize how much you neglect your eye health. Through your everyday activities, you expose your eyes unnecessarily to certain risks, such as irritation, infections, and even vision loss. Here are some important tips for eye care:

## Healthy Eating is the Way:

Remember that everything in excess can be harmful. Avoid excessive use of fried foods, salt, sugar, and red meat. Instead, opt for a variety of fruits, vegetables, fresh greens, and nuts. The intake of vitamins, minerals, healthy proteins, omega-3, and lutein is the right path, as antioxidant-rich foods provide strong support for eye health, delaying the onset of diseases such as cataracts and macular degeneration.

## Good Sunglasses Make a Difference:

Excessive unprotected exposure to sunlight can cause many diseases and harm your eye health. To protect yourself from these radiations, it's advisable to use sunscreen daily for your skin and sunglasses with ultraviolet filter lenses. Ophthalmologists recommend that sunglasses should block between 99% and 100% of UVA and UVB rays. Forget about fashion trends and do not choose fake glasses that offer no guarantee in this regard.

## Know Your Family's Health History:

Several eye diseases are hereditary, including myopia, glaucoma, or cataracts, among others. Therefore, it's advisable to talk to your grandparents, parents, and even older siblings to see if they've experienced any eye diseases. If your research yields positive results, it's important to see an ophthalmologist and report the information. Prevention is essential when it comes to eye health.

## Exercise control over your weight

Obesity is certainly a gateway to the development of various diseases. Diabetes, for example, can lead to vision loss in the long run. If you are overweight, you should seek medical help and seriously adopt a food re-education!

## Always wash your hands

Their hands touch everything, so they are responsible for the spread of much of the diseases. A hand contaminated by any communicable disease can spread this disease to many others. So, after any activity where there is use of hands, wash them. Avoid touching, scratching your eyes with dirty hands; this can lead you to contract a disease.

## If you smoke, it is convenient to stop

Smoking compromises the blood circulation of the retina and affects vision at any stage of life. Therefore, it is ideal to stop as soon as possible. This helps reduce the chances of developing cataracts, glaucoma, and age-related macular degeneration. But the best thing is that you didn't even start smoking!

## Your eyes need to rest

Do not overdo it in front of your computer, laptop, tablet or mobile phone. Make a stop every twenty minutes, averting your gaze for about 20 seconds to something far away. It may seem simple, but this measure prevents eye stress, dryness of the eyes, irritation and discomfort of vision. Those who spend a lot of time with their eyes fixed only on what is close, end up having difficulty seeing further.

# 09- HAIR CARE

Whenever I see a young person with poorly maintained hair, I envision an adult who is relaxed about their appearance. This reminds me of a friend who told me more than once, "When I see a woman walking with a man with unkempt hair, I get the impression that she's out with her father or grandfather, not her partner!" I want to clarify here that maintaining your gray hair is optional, but keeping them neglected is plain carelessness!

Given the importance of taking care of your appearance, I'll provide some crucial tips for maintaining and caring for men's hair:

— Absolutely avoid excessive use of hair gel. Excessive gel can cause dryness in your hair, making it brittle. Over time, this leads to an itchy scalp and inevitable hair loss. Use gel only when necessary and in moderation. Don't overdo it!

— If you like wearing caps and hats, use them in moderation. Understand the difference between necessity and choice. Learn to distinguish one from the other and use them appropriately.

— Use a shampoo specifically designed for dandruff. Dandruff is a chronic and congenital condition caused by the production of sebum in the sebaceous glands. It affects men more frequently, and its causes are related to genetic and hormonal factors.

— Wash your hair moderately, and pay attention to the frequency of washing. Always dry your hair gently. Never, under any circumstances, go to bed with wet hair.

— Don't use conditioners indiscriminately. Choose the right conditioner for your hair type. If necessary, consult a dermatologist. Remember, excess of anything can be harmful.

— Keep your beard and hair well-groomed. Well-maintained hair and a neatly trimmed beard will earn you many points with the female population.

— Make a habit of taking good care of your hair. A haircut can not only offer a new look but also restore health to your hair. If you want stronger, more beautiful, and well-maintained hair, regular visits to the barber are essential.

Note:
Every woman loves to run her fingers through a man's hair. Knowing this, give her a good reason to do so. Keep your hair well maintained, to be a flashy. The tip was given!

Be vigilant with your health. Disease not even in a dream! If you get sick, it may seem natural. But, your friends will not be happy to visit you. All friend finds it depressing to visit another who is sick. And do not think ill of any of them. Who promised to stand by their side in health and disease was his wife. Your friend can stand by your side in health

or disease, notice the
difference (in the
pub or at home);
only in the pub
he will miss
you!

# THE SEXUAL ACT AND ITS IMPORTANCE IN MARITAL LIFE

*When it comes to sex, it's not the boldest
who take the first step; they are merely
facilitators ready to be practical
and not waste time!*
*Della Santa – July 13th, 2020*

I often say that sex, during an active period (and let's be clear about this), is an indicator of whether a couple is doing well or not. So, if you notice that sex is lacking, you need to seek and discover what is causing it. Sexual inactivity can happen, but it is temporary. If it persists, something is definitely wrong, either on one side or the other, or even on both. So, without blaming yourself or the other side, look for a solution. If there is a lack of affection, attention, or focus on the other, try to provide it. If you see the other person distancing themselves, try to see what you are doing wrong, perhaps not necessarily wrong, but contradictory. It's common and natural to think that you're pleasing, but in reality, you might be displeasing. So, seek solutions. There's no magic, but there are actions. A trip, a vacation, enjoying something different together without thinking in advance, "She won't like it." If it's something new, even better. What we've never done can make us apprehensive at first, but after the initial moment, it becomes charming, a unique pleasure, different from the usual, and this marks positively. However, you might tell me, as many people do, "I don't have the time or money to play around!" I would say that life is about choices, and you are making a choice. I've seen many successful individuals who don't enjoy going home. This is because they believe that home is a hell. Well, your home, your sanctuary, was a choice and was what you wanted most. If you chose wrong, then you'll need patience. If everything were exactly the way we wanted, nobody would do anything; everyone would want to laze around, even the silliest of the silly! So, my friend, fight for it, do your part! Here, I want to make it clear that doing your part means "doing what is given to you as an obligation or not and making the other person's life easier!" Was I clear? Did you understand? If not, let me explain: you need to do much more than a normal man does. Normal is anyone else; not you. You are a super husband, a super worker, a super father, a super companion, and a super friend. You are all of that, buddy! Does it sound strange? Well, don't think so. That's how your wife sees you. She didn't choose you by chance. She chose you! Ah, and if you haven't shacking up with her yet, rest assured that this is exactly how she will see you! Accept it if you're sure that's what you want, or cut the line if you find it impossible to live with this pure reality! However, I want to leave a reminder here: every rule has an exception. And for sure, this one is and will never be different! As I initially discussed the importance of sex in a relationship, I can't close this topic without mentioning some little things that can influence, depending on each person's temperament and taste, positively or negatively in a couple's sexual life. Here are some points:

— Don't focus on pornography, don't pay attention to what the actors and actresses do in their scenes. They are not there to show the true reality of sex but an unsustainable fantasy for normal standards. So, don't apply what they do in your bedroom with your partner. If you both agree and she wants to try something, then do it. But don't be deluded; this is not a routine for a couple. If you insist on this subject, the decline, at least in your performance, will be steep!

— Your woman has the attributes you know. You don't need to keep checking if her breasts are perky, if her buttocks are firm, if her waist is slim. She's your woman, the one you met and chose, and she's changing over time, just like you. If you have to look, let it be for a new dress, a skirt, or pants she's wearing, not for her body! This will undermine the relationship because she will think your gaze is a negative critique. But in any case, if you have to look, let it be with eyes of desire. That way, your woman will adore it!

— Respect anatomy. Your woman doesn't have to be like those in the porn industry, just as you don't have to be like a gigolo. Private parts are different, nipples are different, legs are different. The body is different, both in anatomy and sexual stimulation. Some shave, some don't. Does it matter? I don't think so. What truly matters is character!

— If once is enough, there's no reason for two... Fancy drugs might be good for the moment; they will give you the feeling of prolonging the act, perhaps pleasure, here and now; but later, they will turn into torment! Is it worth it? Think about it before resorting to this option.

— Every man greatly values his tool, his penis. But it's common to see men with low self-esteem because of their manhood. Of course, there's always someone who puts certain myths in the heads of those who prefer not to think, not to analyze things; I'd say they have some strange ideas. And then, they turn to the guy and tell him that women like a big penis. But, will it be? Let's think for a moment... If you can bring a woman to orgasm using an eight-centimeter finger or a tongue of the same size, why does your penis have to be big? Based on this, my friend, it's better to know how to use it! If you do it well, everything will work out, and that's the end of it! One thing you can be sure of is that if your tool is big and you don't know how to use it, most of the time, you'll be left high and dry. I'm saying this because I know that, for a man to experience total satisfaction, he needs conviction; he needs to believe wholeheartedly that he's satisfying someone. And of course, I'm talking about someone who is yours, your partner, and someone you want to give your best to! Was I clear? Well... Understand that size isn't identity, ok!

— A woman's moan during a sexual encounter doesn't necessarily mean she's loving it, and the absence of a moan doesn't determine that she's not enjoying it. In fact, those who think that a woman needs to moan like she's in distress to make it clear that the sex is very enjoyable are mistaken. Generally, the moans are light, very low, so as not to attract the attention of eavesdroppers. Some women can't tune out the noises around them, so they remain quieter and let their breathing become more pronounced as they reach ecstasy. So, forget the screaming, the shouting that is often expected. If you have some experience with good sexual relationships, you might have already realized that reality is different. In porn movies, it's one thing; in our real world, it's different. And please, don't try to perform like the professionals in the porn industry, unless she asks you to. If you're interested in doing so and you're unsure if she wants it or not, ask if it's alright, give her a hint of what you want, observe her expressions to be sure if they're of pleasure or disgust. If she indicates that it's okay and she wants more, go ahead and take the lead!

If you're interested in a girl, forget about certain details like shaving, wearing lipstick, painted nails, brushed hair, etc. If you're going to pay attention, it should be to her receptivity, to her feminine way of dealing with the masculine side; whether she's receptive or not. Often, women didn't have time to shave. In the rush, their nails weren't done, and their hair wasn't brushed. What she really needed at that moment was to be present at the event or ended up there by mere chance. But it's also her right; in case she doesn't like any of that, she prefers to be simple, "Au naturel," as a friend of mine would say.

Once, and it was nice, I met a woman who attracted me immensely. When we got into bed, I was surprised by a pubic area that looked more like a forest. In our conversation, she noticed I was taken aback and explained to me that in the land she came from, women didn't usually shave as a protective measure. It was part of their culture. I accepted it, especially because she appeared very feminine and extremely clean! It was a valuable experience, and I want to emphasize that it's the way to go!

— If you're into unconventional sex, take it slow. Some women like it, but not all. For example, some women love oral sex, and some detest it. As for anal sex, for many, it's out of the question! But for others, it's a matter of conquest; meaning, you need to win them over. Pay attention to one detail: **con-quer**! Conquering is not grabbing, taking something from someone who doesn't want to give it to you. Conquering is being gentle and patient, using kind words, convincing arguments, and, above all, actions that please. In the name of pleasure in bed or in the 'matel[8],' you can do anything as long as you know how to get what you want!

— Liking or not liking, that is the question. If this expression sounds strange to you, don't worry because I'll explain. In the sexual act between a man and a woman, there is always a moment called the 'culminating point of the act,' the moment of climax. It's also at this time that one

---

[8] In the bush.

or the other loses touch with reality and ends up doing things that are considered outside the norm. For example, some women like to be called "my little slut," "your bitch," "naughty girl," "slut," "bitch," etc. And others even like to get some slaps that, according to some reports, enhance pleasure. Well, in the same line, there are men with their masculine eccentricities that aren't very different. They often like to be called "my man," "my stallion," "you naughty," "shameless," and so on. However, I would say you need to be careful adopting this kind of behavior because not everyone likes it. It's advisable to have a conversation beforehand to avoid any mishaps or even provoke a "performance issue" at the crucial moment. If you don't like profanity, hearing a swear word during the act can spoil it for you. But understand that it can also happen with your partner.

Once, a friend of mine told me the following story: "I went out with a woman, and after a few drinks, we decided to have sex. We ended up at a motel and went for it. At one point, she gave me a couple of punches in the lower back, saying the following: 'You son of a bitch, you made me climax!' He finished the story by telling me that he felt attacked because he was left speechless by the punches and then had to hear that his mother was a whore. Can you believe it? Honestly, I believe that after something like that, any normal individual is a candidate for performance issues, and he told me he had one! Now, just to add: for a man, if he has performance issues, it's visible; for a woman, you need to notice it or hear it from her; but there are many who don't say anything. But the truth is they leave frustrated. This should not and must not happen. But as I said at the beginning, everything is valid as long as it's agreed upon in advance. For a couple, everything that is good needs to be mutual; it can't be good for just one!

— Be a little bit perverted. For example, know how to go down on a woman. There are women who like men like that. In fact, there are women who only experience pleasure with men like that. But, to put things calmly and gently, it's essential to know that there are women who like sex much more than men, and for this type of woman, the man is never considered perverted. He is just someone striving to give his best to his female partner. But, to do this, he first needs to discover what she likes. We're talking about women, and they are not all the same. It's up to you to discover what your partner likes. Here's a tip: some women enjoy to suck the man, but they don't like to be sucked by him. Perhaps they lack confidence, perhaps they've been through some disappointment, which also happens with men. Nevertheless, taking it easy, you really should try to find out, give it a shot; you might end up doing it well, and she'll love it. To perform oral sex properly, you need to have class and some knowledge. Otherwise, you'll end up spoiling what could be a beautiful moment in the relationship. But, if you do it right, if you make her enjoy it, she'll want more and more. Then, it's up to you; work on improving your performance!

— Make lovemaking a moment of pure pleasure. Never make love as if the world were about to end. You can take a woman, lean her against the wall, push her onto the bed, jump on top of her, take her up on the counter, throw her on the table, but remember: you're dealing with a human being made of flesh and blood, with feelings and everything else. So, don't hurt her, don't leave marks. If you want to leave your mark, give her a passionate fuck, but add tenderness; that's what matters! She will remember the tenderness you showed her much more than the physical mark you left.

Remember to be attentive; some women are naturally aroused. An important detail is to keep an eye on her eyes and what she observes in you. This may not seem like much, but some women get wet just by looking at the bulge in a man's pants. Once, a woman told me that when she's interested in a guy, he just needs to come over and take her because she's already prepared for him. From there, if the woman is signaling that she wants you, let her take the lead, follow her lead... or don't go if you're not interested. Just as she's not obligated to want you, you have no obligation to want her either!

Men are easily fooled; that's well-known, but so are women. What not everyone knows is that one illusion replaces another, but it doesn't erase disappointments. Disappointment, if you have it, learn to live with it and move on with life. Some days you win, others you lose. Winning and losing are part of life in its various aspects!

And to conclude, I leave you with the following verse for your reflection:

*An honorable man honors the woman.*
*A man without a woman*
*is a boat without a rudder,*
*a path without direction.*
*He is a wanderer,*
*without stopped*
*defined!*

The end

# BIBLIOGRAPHY


PEREIRA, Flávio A. Modern Sexual Encyclopedia, Vol. 1, 2, 3. São Paulo: Libra Empresa Editorial Ltda, 1971.

Marcela Lemos, on May 27, 2020. Testosterone. Available at > https://www.tuasaude.com < Accessed on 07/13/2020.

https://medprev.online/blog/exams-every-man-should-take.html - Accessed on 07/12/2020.

www.laboratorioexame.com.br - Accessed on 07/12/2020.

www.santapaula.com.br - Accessed on 07/11/2020.

www.minhavida.com.br - Accessed on 07/11/2020.

www.minutosaudadavel.com.br - Accessed on 07/10/2020.

www.tuasaude.com.br - Accessed on 07/10/2020.

www.tudosbrefigado.com.br - Accessed on 07/10/2020.

# COMMENTS RECEIVED FROM READERS

## COMMENT 01

By: Pedro de Oliveira

Your new book: "From Man to Men."

Speaking about Aniel dos Santos, a fellow of ACLAV and a prolific and forward-thinking writer, is easy for me, as I have known him since childhood. Aniel has always been ahead of his time, at the forefront, at the top of the cultural and intellectual hierarchy. While the rest of us struggled to speak Portuguese, Aniel was already dabbling in English and Spanish; he learned by watching movies at Cine São Geraldo. Despite a childhood marked by difficulties (our childhoods were like that), he managed to turn things around and do things that were far from ordinary for us, his friends from the neighborhood. He knew where he wanted to go and sought his place in the sun. This is how he studied, went to college, worked until he retired, and dedicated himself to many important things. The same goes for his life as a writer. He writes things that are different, unconventional, and he's not ashamed to be happy, to speak his mind, and tell people how he thinks, whether they agree or not. His first published book received high praise from our patron, Dr. Petrônio Brás. He has already written more than 15 works. Now he is launching "From Man to Men," which could also be "From Man to Women," in this book where he provides good tips and advice for a man's daily life and his marital relationships (or relationships). Aniel innovates by using the pseudonym M. GEESCOGE. He says, "This book proposes to guide men in their relationships with women, whether at the beginning or in a relationship that has some history. These guidelines are the result of observations in everyday life and stories from simple, straightforward people, often in moments of confession, but with a touch of humor. It also addresses concerns about men's health, with tips for staying in shape and not failing in dealing with women. In short, this is a book that should be part of your daily life and, why not, your bedside book? So, in a clever, smart way, Aniel gives us a message, to succeed with your wife and other women, why use Viagra? Read and be happy.

Comment posted on Facebook by Pedro de Oliveira, writer, and academic of the Academies of Letters ACLAV and ACLECIA.


## COMMENT 02

By: Adão Rafael Morais

Humbly, you were born to feed the less fortunate and those deprived of knowledge with your culture. I am pleased to know that you are fulfilled with your mission: to be useful. Having the recognition of a colleague of the same caliber is gratifying. Everything he said about you is not news to me. The first time, without even knowing me, you served cold juice to my friends and a cowboy whiskey to me, and this happened on a scorching sunny afternoon. At that moment, I realized that you had something different. My innocence in not being able to define what I really wanted at that moment made you assertive. I told this story to several people, and I even used it in a meeting with colleagues. I can say that I learned from you. You are a man of many strengths, skillful with words, and have the power of persuasion. "From Man to Men" is just a sample of your potential. I tip my hat to you and thank you for being my friend. Thank you!

## COMMENT 03

By: Jaíba

## About the Book "From Man to Men"

As a great thinker, who eloquently and wisely expresses his opinions, I am dazzled by how simply this book has been presented, poetically, exposing his thoughts on everyday facts, sometimes ordinary but putting us in the spotlight when we encounter them in our daily lives. A book to be read and reread, making the most of the content, which is very good and interesting. My sincere congratulations...

Edson Elias Vitor (Jaíba)
June 7th, 2021

******

# WORK OF THE AUTHOR (Portuguese)

— Footsteps. (poems 1982).

— The Great Race. (short stories 1982).

— Marathons. (poems from 1983).

— Diversities. (various writings 1985).

— No Extremes. (poems 1986).

— Children of Destiny. (Romance 1988).

— Only Just for You. (thoughts 1989).

— A Dose of Laughter. (jokes and anecdotes 1989).

— Tales That I Tell. (short stories 1990).

— Extraordinary Raw Material Control Applied in Reduction Furnaces. (Monograph 1998).

— Calm. (thoughts 2000).

— The player. (novel 2004).

— From Man to Men. — Tips and Cases to Man Knowing and Understanding Women Better. (2019 – English and Portuguese).

— Learning from Life — My Thought for Your Reflection. (2020) About us.

— The New Square Case. (Romance 2022)

# PARTICIPATIONS

01 Poetic anthology of the 50th anniversary of Várzea da Palma, MG, Brazil. (Poems 2003).

02 Poetic Encounter I (Poetry 2007).

03 Poetic Encounter III (Poetry 2015)

04 Poetic anthology of the ACLAV Academy of Sciences, Arts and Letters of Várzea da Palma, MG. (2016).

www.ingramcontent.com/pod-product-compliance
Lightning Source LLC
Chambersburg PA
CBHW070811260726
48660CB00005B/1806